Cory Everson's
FAT-FREE & FIT

Cory Everson's
FAT-FREE & FIT

A Complete Program for Fitness, Exercise,
and Healthy Living

Cory Everson
and Carole Jacobs

Photography by Robert Reiff

A Perigee Book

Before beginning any dietary or exercise program, always consult with your doctor. The exercises in this book are intended only for healthy people. People with health problems should not follow these routines without a physician's approval.

Perigee Books
are published by
The Berkley Publishing Group
200 Madison Avenue
New York, NY 10016

Library of Congress Cataloging-in-Publication Data
Everson, Cory.
  [Fat-free & fit]
  Cory Everson's Fat-free & fit : a complete program for fitness, exercise, and healthy living / by Cory Everson and Carole Jacobs ; photography by Robert Reiff.
    p. cm.
  ISBN 0-399-51858-4 (acid-free paper)
  1. Physical fitness for women. 2. Exercise for women. 3. Women—Nutrition.
I. Jacobs, Carole. II. Title. III. Title: Fat-free & fit.
RA778.E927 1994   93-36944 CIP
613.7′045—dc20

Cover design by Mike Stromberg
Cover photograph © by Robert Reiff

Printed in the United States of America
   3 4 5 6 7 8 9 10

Acknowledgments

To Steve Delsohn and Frank Weimann at the Literary Group: The greatest book agents in the entire world and the reason this book became reality.

To Carole Jacobs: When Carole came into my life and joined efforts with me in this book, I got more than a talented coauthor. I got a close, sincere, loving friend. Carole, this is just the beginning. Thanks!

To my best friends, Michelle LeMay, Cameo Kneuer, and Charlie Lindsey, three people I would never be able to live without!

To my little old German Dad, "Papm," who helps me invent and cook non-fat recipes and listens with an open heart to his occasionally crazed daughter's problems.

To "MooMoo" (Mom), who has been the most incredible, strong, effervescent, charming, and giving role model any daughter could ever hope to have.

And to the rest of my family, who will never quite realize the true extent of my love and need for every one of them. Because of them, I am the luckiest person on earth!

To Kimberly Ex, my magical makeup artist and friend, who has such talent that she can make me look great even when to myself, I look like a haggard, swollen pufferfish that should be put out of its misery and used for shark bait.

To my ex-husband, Jeff Everson, who will always be a huge part of my life and everything I do and am—no matter what!

To "Schtoy Boy," Stevie Donia, who rescued me by being my very strength through the toughest time of my life, and with his unlimited emotional support, understanding, and unconditional love kept me afloat. For that I will always be grateful, and never be able to thank him enough. I love ya Bollér.

To the real loves of my life, Baby Bolaro, Billy Boy, and White Guy, my beloved pets, whom I would honestly die for.

To Deke Anderson, a.k.a. "Deedle Doy Dumpster," or "Mr. Smart Guy," for your absolute generosity in helping to make my work easier with your optimism and giving and for lifting my spirits with your exaggerated rubber face expressions and contorted awful looks of horrid agony, as demonstrated throughout this book. You are truly a watering hole!

To Robert Reiff, not only one of the best photographers in the world but one of the best life-long friends a person could wish to have. Thanks for being so many things to me.

To Joe Weider, who probably has no clue how much I love and admire him and crave the way he treats me like a dad would. Papa Joe . . . you fill a very special need in me.

Finally, to all my wonderful fans, who continue to bless me with their love and support and keep me motivated, creative, and most of all, happy.

I love you all!
Cory Everson

Contents

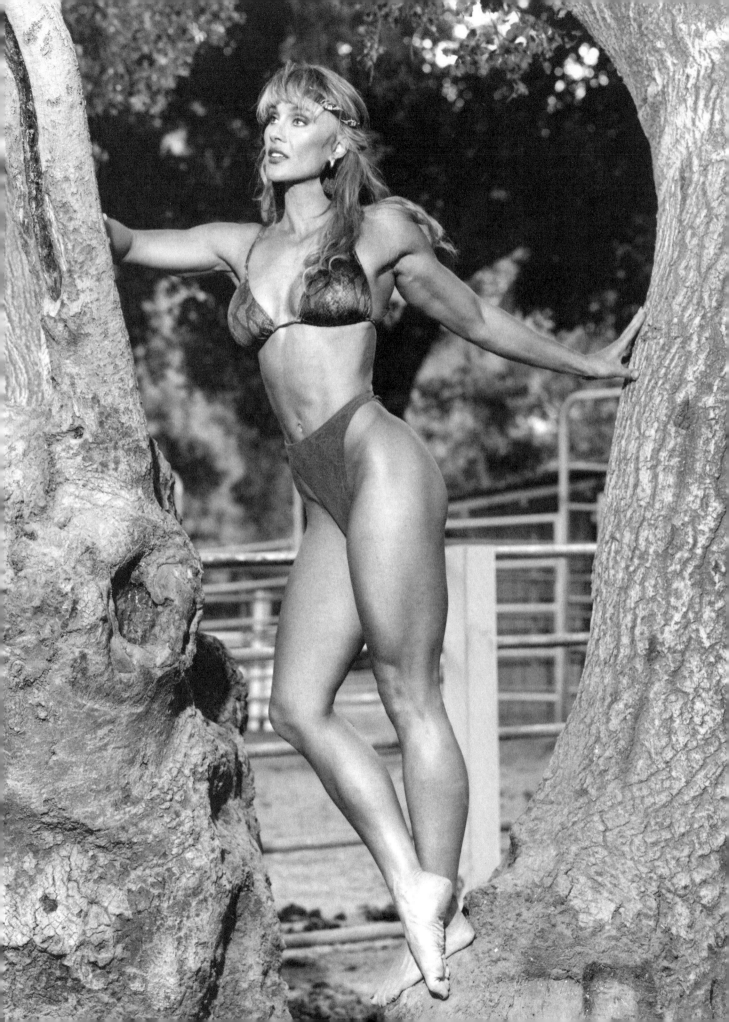

Introduction

A Body to Live For—Not to Die For

I know what you're thinking. What would somebody like Cory Everson know about fat? She doesn't have any, does she? Besides, didn't I read somewhere that all those women bodybuilders work out 19 hours a day and live on rice cakes? How can I possibly look like her and have a life? Or at least a life that doesn't revolve around the gym?

Okay, ladies, let's set the record straight. Now I'd be the first to admit that I didn't become Ms. Olympia six years in a row by resting on my laurels—or anything else, for that matter.

During that time, maintaining a championship build was my full-time job. When you're banking on your physique, you can't afford to let your bottom line go to pot or your bank account could do likewise.

But I'll let you in on a little secret. I've never been as happy with my life and body as I am today. While I loved every minute of it, those six years of nonstop professional competition, with their draining training schedule, ultrastrict nutrition regimen, and hectic travel schedule, really took their toll.

Granted, I wouldn't win any bodybuilding titles today because my muscles are too small. But my proportions are exactly the same as they were in my competing days, and my increased body fat is evenly distributed to give me a soft, feminine look. My hair is shinier, my skin has a new glow, and for the first time in six years I can focus on something besides my biceps—my painting and acting, for instance—or the simple pleasure of a sunset or a visit to a batting cage.

If someone tried to tell me three years ago when I left professional bodybuilding that fitness would be this easy today, I probably would have laughed. If you want the truth, I was scared to death to quit! I was afraid that once I stopped working out 20 hours a day and started eating more normally, I'd blow up like the Goodyear Blimp. I couldn't imagine maintaining a firm bottom line if I was going to be sitting on it all day in front of an easel. Maybe I wouldn't become a famous artist, but I'd probably become a fat one.

Then I read somewhere that muscle has memory and that even when you're not training hard your body will remember how to maintain its shape. It sounded like thigh in the sky to me. Three years later, I'm writing this book to tell you it's true—and to show you how easy it is to get in shape, regardless of the body you have now.

We're not going to wave any magic wands here. Losing weight and firming up will require effort on your part, but not nearly as much as you might think. In fact, combine a low-fat diet with four hours a week of exercise and you're on your way.

Once you've established new eating and exercise habits and provided your body with

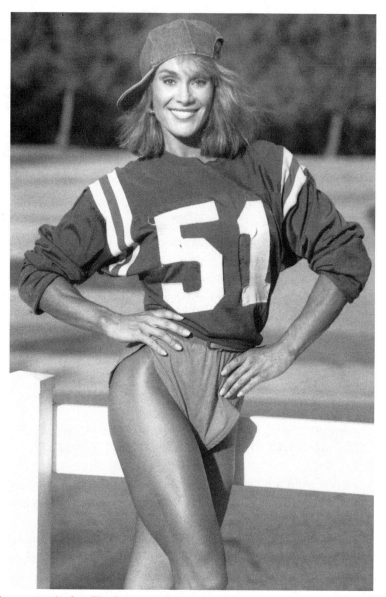

A body to live for, not to die for. That's my *modus operandi.*

"muscle memory," you'll be amazed, as was I, that your body will do everything it can to help you stay there. Getting out of shape will take work on your part. Eating dessert three nights in a row or even missing a week's worth of workouts won't make a dent once you've given your body a healthy blueprint to follow.

In fact, there are days and even entire weeks when I'm too busy to exercise or even fix a real meal. One day a friend came over for lunch and the only thing in my refrigerator was bird food for my parrots. As far as pumping heavy iron, the only heavyweight in my life these days is Mr. Beaver, my pet, pot-bellied pig. Speedwalking and light weight training keep me in shape, and my mirror and my favorite jeans are all I need to "measure" my progress. If my cheeks don't look like a chipmunk's and my jeans zip without a struggle, I know I'm within my "safe" weight range.

The goal of this program is to provide a healthful diet and exercise program you can maintain on a day-to-day basis without sacrificing your life for it.

Take a good look at yourself in the mirror. I'm built like a dumbbell—wide on both ends and thin in the middle. If you're a large woman with a big frame, you're never going to look fragile; if you're a very petite woman, you're probably never going to look like those Russian swimmers who look as if they're built to remain standing through an atom bomb blast.

My goal in writing this book is not to give you a body to die for, but a body to live for—in other words, the very best version of you.

I'm not going to promise that you'll wind up looking like a runway model. I could live on bird food for the rest of my life and never be that thin, nor would I want to be.

But give this program a try, and within three months, you will find yourself standing in front of a mirror saying, "Wow! I never knew I could look this good!"

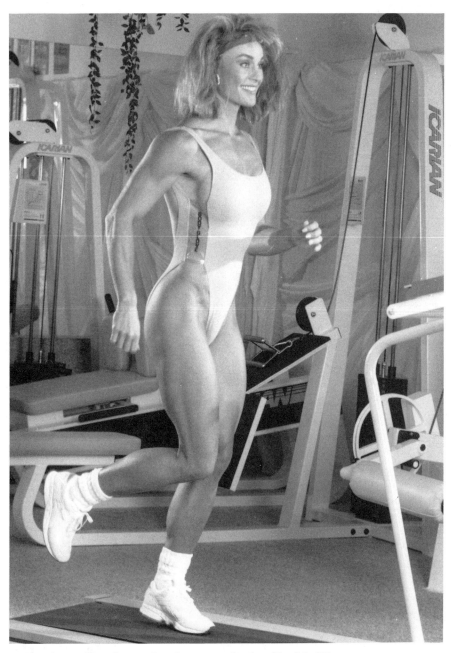

Here I am today, just as fit as I was when I was a professional bodybuilder.

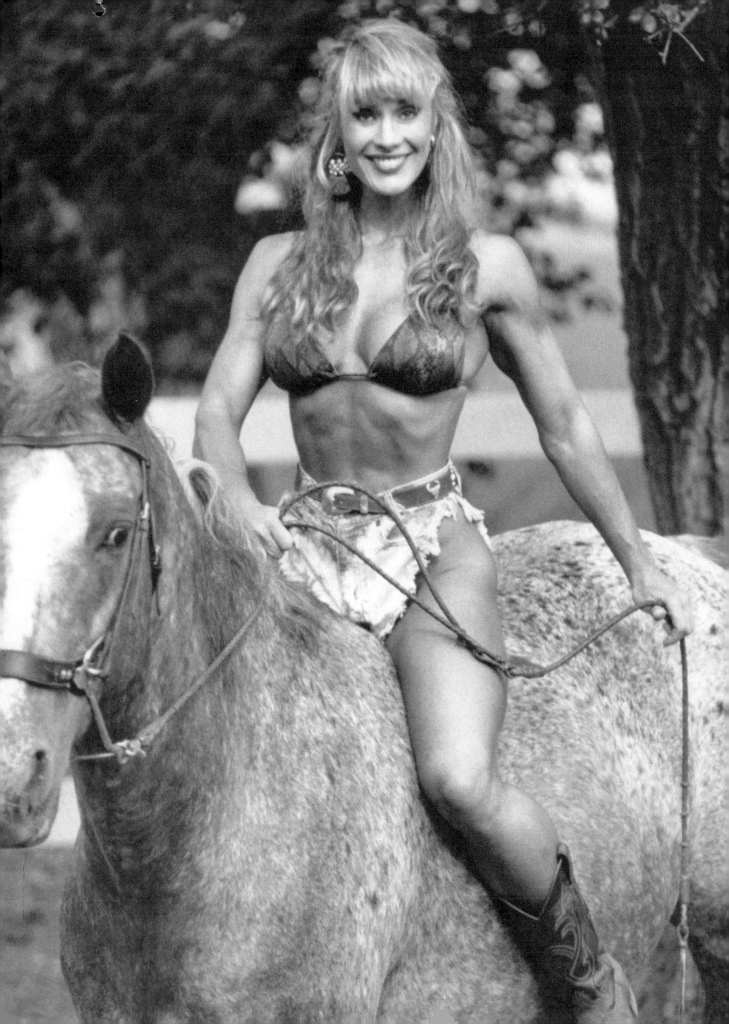

One

Diet Is a Four-Letter Word

If anyone has the skinny on fat, it's female bodybuilders. They live in a world where killer quads and pie-in-the-sky thighs are *de rigueur,* and where a quivering bottom can doom their careers.

Long before Americans started getting wise to the benefits of low-fat living, it was a way of life for female bodybuilders like me. My personal trainer, Jeff, was a regular part of my life—and believe me, he got pretty darn personal. If I had an extra jiggle or ounce of fat that might disqualify me from winning a title, he found it.

Not that I didn't appreciate his hawk-eyed monitoring. Bodybuilding was, after all, my bread and butter for almost eight years. We both knew that if I got too flabby, my bank account would get too skinny.

Meanwhile, finding ways to maintain a prize-winning physique without sacrificing my health was a constant struggle and delicate balancing act. Not only did I have to maintain a very low body fat but I also had to stay strong and healthy to compete. The rigors of constant travel and inhuman amounts of exercise—four to six hours a day—meant every ounce of food I consumed had to be power-packed for maximum nutrition and performance. Chocolate bars? Only in my dreams.

To survive the muscle-bound fast lane required the equivalent of a Ph.D. in nutrition and exercise science. In the course of nearly a decade-long bodybuilding career, I talked to every fat expert I could find. Unfortunately, back then, the experts lacked the sophisticated knowledge we have today concerning fat and metabolism. Much of my training was trial and error, and I made a lot of mistakes on the way to becoming a championship bodybuilder.

For starters, I worked out too much and ate too little in relation to my energy needs and metabolic burn. I can still remember my mother waving my dinner plate at me as I rushed out the door to go running. If I knew then what I know now about nutrition and exercise, I could have saved myself hours of obsessive workouts and would have eaten a lot more. What you'll learn about fat in this book comes from my years of interaction with fat specialists–from the training partners who helped me win the Ms. Olympia contest six times in a row, to those who helped me redefine my exercise and diet program so I could maintain a slim physique while living a more sedentary lifestyle.

The diet and exercise programs we describe in this book won't necessarily give you the body of a fashion model–to do so I'd have to lose most of my muscle, which is taboo in my book–and in this book, too.

Rather than a body to die for, we want to give you a healthy, attractive balance of lean body mass and muscle tone. In other words, a body to live, for and the very best version of you.

DIET IS A FOUR-LETTER WORD

Let's start the program with a discussion of the ultimate four-letter word: DIET. You eat like a bird but look like a blimp? I believe you. If fat is a four-letter word, dieting is the curse that gets us there. Think of your metabolism as a furnace. Dieting progressively lowers your metabolism until it's more of a flicker than a fat-burning flame.

And studies show that most fat people don't overeat; they undereat and subsequently retrain their bodies to perform on less fuel, according to nutrition expert Marc Sorenson, Ed.D., author of the book *Megahealth* (National Institute of Fitness, 1992) and co-owner of the National Institute of Fitness (NIF) in Ivins, Utah, a fitness center where obese clients lose hundreds of pounds and keep them off permanently by following a low-fat diet and a daily walking program.

Sorenson says chronic dieters not only burn 700 fewer calories a day but regain 18 times more fat on the same number of calories as nondieters. The result is that they become heavier– and "fatter"–with each attempted diet.

According to fat guru Martin Katahn, Ph.D., former director of the weight-loss clinic at Vanderbilt University in Nashville, Tennessee, author of several books on low-fat eating and the man who demystified metabolism for the masses (Katahn made "set point theory" a household phrase), if being overweight was merely a matter of vanity, we could probably all put up with the extra jiggle and bounce. But excess fat is more than the stuff that comes between us and our favorite jeans; it's dangerous stuff–the leading culprit in heart disease and many forms of cancer, including many types that specifically afflict women, including breast cancer. Fat, in fact, has killed more people than the atom bomb. Any way you measure it, excess fat is an explosive issue.

NO FUN BEING FAT

Check out any magazine cover: Our society has an addiction to thinness. Thin is in; fat is taboo.

Overweight and obese people often suffer from societal stigmas that prevent them from getting jobs, promotions, or being viewed as worthwhile human beings. According to a series in the *New York Times* on "Fat in America," fat people are often subjected to cruel and inhumane treatment by employers, strangers–even physicians who refuse to treat them and consider them disgusting. If you've ever seen an obese person eating in a restaurant, you know what I mean. It's not unusual for people to stare at them or even walk by their table to see if they've ordered enormous portions. In most cases, they eat normally and are overweight because of genetics.

Scientists are also guilty of bias, blaming the obese for their inability to keep lost weight off when in fact their genes are against them.

A recent study of formerly obese people who lost weight through intestinal bypass surgery revealed that they would rather be deaf, blind, or have a leg amputated than be fat again. Being too fat not only lowers our self-esteem but sometimes our status and our earning potential, too.

FATTER THAN EVER

Now that low-fat is the buzzword of the best-seller list, you'd think we'd be a nation of skinny women. But statistics show we're not only getting fatter but we are resorting to accursed crash dieting in unprecedented droves. Last year, more than 25 million women voluntarily starved themselves on diets doomed to boomerang. Are you one of them?

Of course, there's a flip side. Sometimes, the urge to be thin is so powerful that many otherwise logical women wander over the dietary deep end and into eating disorders, inviting metabolic ruin where the fat they temporarily lose is insignificant compared to their other losses—their hair, teeth, menstrual periods, bone density—sometimes even their lives. We'll look more at eating disorders and its twin obsession, exercise abuse, in Chapter 10.

OUR LOVE-HATE RELATIONSHIP WITH FAT

Let's take a closer look at this thing called fat. We loathe it because it jiggles when we walk, pads our curves, and endangers our health. But we also love it because it tastes good and because we have an inherited preference for fatty foods dating back to prehistoric days, when eating excess fat ensured we'd survive long enough to reproduce.

Remember Cave Woman Jane? Her high-fat diet enabled her to stay warm in those cold caves so she could reproduce the species. And let's face it, girls, without Jane's preference for fat, we wouldn't be here today. With her big hips, thunder thighs, and ample bosom, Jane was the femme fatale of the cave scene—a "body beautiful" that prevailed until the flat-chested, knobby-kneed, Twiggy-thin flappers of the 1920s turned the female body image inside out and spawned a century of fat phobia—and eating disorders that continues to this day.

FRIEND AND FOE

Besides, fat's not all bad. According to Katahn, while too much fat is the leading cause of heart disease, diabetes, and many female cancers, we all need to eat and wear a little fat to stay healthy.

Fat cushions our internal organs and is necessary to dissolve some of the vitamins we consume in food. It also provides bodily warmth so we don't freeze in winter or in air-conditioned buildings and gives us smooth, soft skin and shiny hair.

A little fat can even help keep us youthful-looking; women over 40 are often encouraged to gain a few pounds to plump out facial wrinkles. Without any fat, we'd look like scrawny chickens—old beyond our years with skin like dried-out leather and hair like straw.

By skimping on dietary fat, we also sabotage our body's ability to absorb essential, fat-soluble vitamins (such as E) and many fat-soluble minerals, which in turn could lead to a host of mental and physical problems, including depression, skin problems, and malnutrition.

Finally, women who overly skimp on fat often lose their menstrual periods—sometimes for months or years—and may jeopardize their chance for having children, says Larrian Gillespie, M.D., a Beverly Hills urologist who specializes in women's disorders.

When I was competing, I often lost my period except for twice a year—Thanksgiving and Christmas. Why? Because I ate more and exercised less during the holidays and my hormonal cycles bounced back to normal.

"Show me a lady eating too little fat and I'll show you a lady who is a ticking time bomb for everything from eating disorders and osteoporosis to troubles during pregnancy or with her female organs," Gillespie says.

So how much fat does a modern-day Jane need for health? According to the United States Department of Agriculture's new Food Guide Pyramid, (see Chapter 4 for details), the ideal diet contains 20 to 30 percent calories from fat. If you consume 1,500 calories a day, that means that at least 300 calories should come from fat.

TOO MUCH OF A GOOD THING

But let's get back to the modern-day fat issue; that is, too much of a good thing. If diets really worked—any diet—we wouldn't have written this book, and you wouldn't have bought it, Despite the diet craze, and there are thousands of diet plans out there, as a population we're becoming increasingly fatter. Between 1963 and 1980, America experienced a 54 percent increase in the rate of obesity among children, and nearly a doubling of superobesity—although children ate slightly fewer calories than in 1963. So if food wasn't making them fatter, what was?

You guessed it: Diets. Obesity is not caused by overeating or eating too many calories, but by eating too much fat, not exercising, and going on repeated diets—which may foster eating disorders because women panic at gaining weight, then starve themselves to lose it. I've seen this happen with professional athletes, models, doctor's wives, and some of the most public, popular celebrities in movies and television. No one is immune. What you see on the outside often comes from a long line of destruction on the inside.

Studies show that women who eat less will ultimately have a higher percentage of body fat than those who eat more—which explains why 40 percent of the women in the U.S. today are overweight.

HOW TO FATTEN A HOG

Want a live version of Porky Pig? Starve 'em! A farmer Sorenson knows claims that the classic method for fattening a hog is to restrict the amount of food they receive for several days until they're so hungry they're squealing. Then the hogs are fed freely for a few days until the process is repeated. The result is a pig who's fat enough to win any blue ribbon. My pet pig, Beaver, by the way, is a consummate grazer like me; his low-fat diet keeps him lean and trim, and he has six straight Mr. Hog-Olympia victories to prove it.

Studies show women who eat 410 fewer calories per day than nondieters also burn 620 fewer calories, becoming increasingly heavier.

In fact, one study of temporarily thinner people showed they burned much fewer calories than nondieters. When they tried to resume their normal diets, they regained an extra eight pounds in 35 days.

NUTS AND BOLTS OF METABOLISM

The fact is, those who diet can truly eat like birds and gain weight on the same number of calories, or even fewer, than nondieters eat to maintain a normal weight. This is because dieting lowers our metabolism, or heat-burning furnace. Our bodies were built to last through thick or thin, feast or famine, and our metabolism is conditioned to burn hot or slow depending on available food resources.

Every time you go on a diet, you lower your metabolism a little more. Within one or two days, your metabolic rate can decrease by 15 to 30 percent because your body senses starvation and resolves to slow down bodily processes to conserve energy to preserve life for the longest time possible.

When you try to resume normal eating habits, your body, which has become accustomed to less, stores the extra calories as fat. The result is that you gain weight—typically about five percent after each diet attempt. Remember what happened to Oprah? Enough said.

The short-term visual and psychological changes keep women coming back to those unhealthy patterns. Just because you lost four pounds by starving yourself doesn't mean starving "works." It only works against you.

DIETS REDUCE MUSCLE

When you lose weight through dieting, part of it is lean tissue—or dense muscle which weighs more than fat and thus burns more calories as you move around. But when you regain weight, you gain it back primarily as fat, which is lighter and requires fewer calories to maintain.

The result is that even if you weigh less, you may have a higher percentage of fat—or get "fatter" as you get thinner.

In one research study, rats were starved to 80 percent of their normal weight. When allowed to eat freely, they ate slightly less than their free-feeding littermates but gained weight 18 times faster!

PERILS OF YO-YO DIETING

If one diet is a problem, a series is a disaster, says Sorenson. He sees it all the time with his clients at NIF. "Some of them are gaining weight on 300 calories a day—or what you'd get by eating two slices of bread and an apple."

Each diet progressively lowers your metabolic rate so that you regain weight more rapidly after each diet; low-calorie diets become less and less effective.

In one study, rats on a diet lost weight in 21 days; when allowed to eat normally, they regained it in 46 days. On the next diet, it took them 46 days to lose the same amount of weight, but they regained it in 15 days—three times faster.

Some people inherit a naturally sluggish metabolism, and it also slows with age, or by a half percent a year from age 26 on, which is why people who were thin all their lives suddenly develop a pot belly or big thighs in mid-life.

Eating disorders are another dangerous downside to dieting. Many women anxious to remain model-thin, even though studies show only five percent of women have the genes to do so, embark on fad diets that render them progressively fatter and foster anorexia nervosa, bulimia, and laxative abuse. Top fashion models openly admitted these excesses in *People* magazine.

No matter what your metabolism is now, you can increase it to a normal "high-burning" level in a matter of months by eating a diet low in fat and high in complex carbohydrates and fiber, and by exercising regularly to build fat-burning muscle and increase your overall percentage of muscle. We'll show you how in the following chapters.

THE REAL SKINNY ON PIGGING OUT

Meanwhile, how do the rules apply when you eat the WHOLE thing—as in the whole pizza, the whole bag of M&M peanuts—or lumberjack servings of Christmas dinner?

Does your metabolism crank on high—like a fire to which you've just added dry wood? Or is that wishful thinking?

I love to eat. In fact, I'd rather exercise for a longer period of time for the privilege of wolfing down a giant Snickers bar. But there are days when no amount of exercise can justify my pig outs (especially around PMS time).

It is OKAY to occasionally chow down—but what happens to all those extra calories? For some answers, we went to Nancy Clark, M.S., R.D., author of *Sports Nutrition Guidebook* (Leisure Press, Champaign, IL, 1990), and a sports nutritionist who counsels everyone from weekend to Olympic athletes.

For starters, you'll probably weigh more the morning after—but don't panic! It's not fat but water, says Clark. "When you overeat, you inevitably consume not only sodium, which can retain water, but also a substantial amount of carbohydrates from bread, potato, stuffing, vegetables, desserts, or whatever your vice. Your body stores these extra carbohydrates in your muscles in the form of glycogen. With each ounce of glycogen, you also store about three ounces of water.

If you are a regular exerciser who works out strenuously every day, your muscles may be chronically glycogen-depleted—particularly if you restrict your caloric intake because of a reducing diet.

Thanks to your eating spree, your muscles finally have a chance to refuel their depleted carbohydrate stores, but, unfortunately, they also retain water at the same time. Consequently, the needle on your scale goes up.

Clark says this weight gain is a positive sign that your muscles are well fueled. In fact, athletes who carbo-load on pasta know the subsequent but temporary 2 to 4 pound weight gain indicates they're primed for the event—and raring to go.

But this water-weight gain can ruin your day if you are a scale worshipper. Our advice is to grin and bear it: This weight gain is transient and will go away within a day or two as

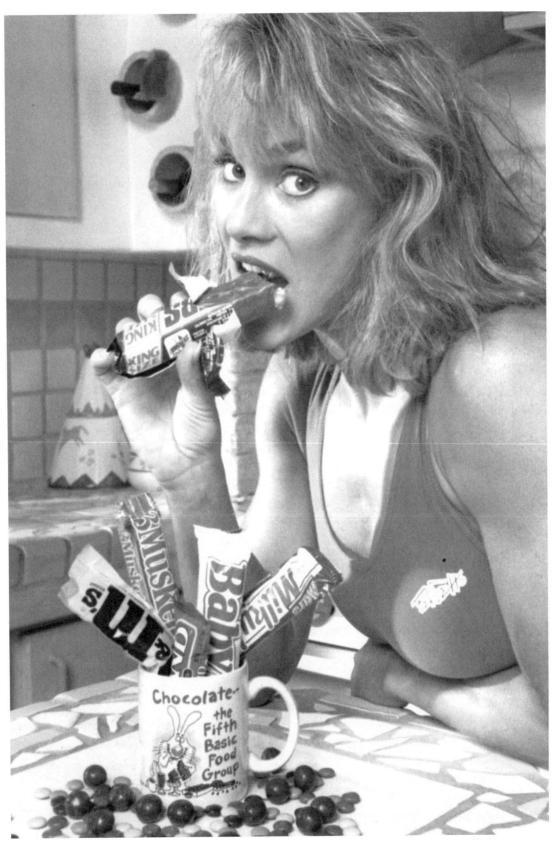

A Snickers a month is my motto. But 24 grams of fat per bar is nothing to snicker at.

you burn off the glycogen during your workouts and excrete other retained fluid. In fact, you may be so energetic during your workout that you may wonder if somebody switched bodies on you in the night.

The downside to overeating is that you have probably eaten excess fat along with the carbs. Your body will quickly store these excess calories as body fat. But before you panic, remember that one pound of fat contains 3,500 excess calories. That's a lot of pie no matter how you slice it, ladies—no mere forkful.

BORN TO GAIN?

Do you seem to gain weight by inhaling apple pie fumes—or by walking past a bakery and peeking at the cream puffs? Me, too! Or so I used to believe until Clark told me otherwise.

Remember, a pound of fat contains 3,500 extra calories—and aromas don't count. However, when a dieter starts to resume normal eating after months of carbohydrate and calorie restrictions, her body clings to water so her chronically depleted glycogen stores can refuel. Consequently, the scale goes up and the dieter feels like a failure who can gain weight on one measly little treat.

The truth is, most of us can pig out one day, undereat the next, and manage to keep our weight on an even keel. This is because Mother Nature does a fine job of regulating body fat within a small range among people who eat appropriately, a phenomena called homeostasis.

Problems with weight gain occur when you pig out consistently—not occasionally. For the most part, people who overindulge on holidays like Thanksgiving will be less hungry the day after and will simply eat less. The body has an amazing ability to maintain a normal weight range if you listen to your appetite and adjust your eating accordingly.

Some people claim they are ravenous the morning after having overeaten. Has my stomach stretched out, they wonder? Not at all. This hunger is due to a blood-sugar imbalance, not a lack of calories, and is totally transient. In fact, it can be easily resolved with a light breakfast, she explains.

FEEDING THE RIGHT HUNGER

Studies show that lean people tend to have a better ability to listen to their appetites than do fatter people, according to Maria Simonson, Ph.D., founder and director of the Health, Stress and Weight Loss Clinic at Johns Hopkins University in Baltimore, Maryland. Generally, they eat when they are hungry and stop when they are content. Overfat people, however, generally eat to fill emotional as well as physical hunger and may continue to feed their face (and figure) long after their stomach has said "enough already!" For instance, people who overeat during stressful periods are overeating for comfort—not hunger—and may even stuff themselves with traditional comfort foods like pudding, mashed potatoes, cookies, cake, or foods that are high in carbohydrates, which tend to have a calming effect, she says.

However, not all bodies respond to pigging out equally. (Sorry, girls, but it's not a fair world.) One woman may eat a whole half gallon of ice cream and gain an ounce; another, a pound. Blame it on heredity, but some people simply gain weight easier and faster than others. Weight is more than just a matter of will power, as research shows.

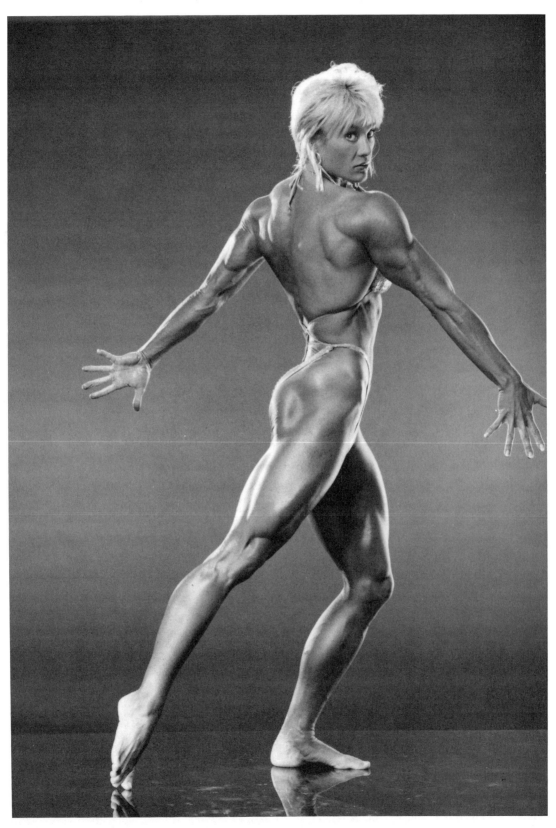

If anyone has the skinny on fat, it's professional bodybuilders, where every ounce of fat you eat is likely to show up sooner or later. (Competition shot 1987)

TWINS IN EVERY SENSE OF THE WORD

In a study of overfeeding reported in the *New England Journal of Medicine* (May 24, 1990) consisting of 12 sets of identical male twins (average age, 21 years old), researchers documented genetic differences in ability to gain weight. Each twin was overfed 1,000 calories per day, 6 days a week for 14 weeks—like eating about two extra Big Macs or 20 Oreo's above and beyond the typical diet—a relatively hard task when repeated day after day. The twins were allowed to walk only 30 minutes per day. Weight gain varied from 9.5 to 29 pounds, with 18 pounds as the average. Although this reflects a wide range of weight gain, each pair of twins responded similarly to the overfeeding. That is, if one twin gained 20 pounds, the other one gained about the same amount.

The bottom line is that genetic factors seem to control one's tendency to deposit body fat, says Clark. If you think that you gain weight easily, take a look at your family members. If you are much leaner than they are, Mother Nature may be trying to fatten you up so you more closely match your inherited body type.

ANATOMY OF A PIG OUT

Let's say you pigged out and ate a half pound of M&M peanuts. Is this like feeding a fire extra logs, which causes it to flare up and burn hotter? In other words, will your metabolism increase to help burn off all those extra calories? Historically, researchers thought yes—and it was nice theory while it lasted. Unfortunately, more current research suggests that gluttony does not significantly boost your metabolism above the cost of handling the calorie load. Nor do you excrete the extra calories in feces. In the overfeeding studies, the subjects flushed about 125 calories per day down the toilet, regardless of their intake. Plain and simple, you store about 60–75 percent of the excess calories as either body fat or muscle tissue. The remaining calories are spent building and maintaining those tissues.

However, when you gain weight, you gain muscle as well as fat. Like fat, muscle can be a storehouse for extra calories. Studies of overweight people show that with a weight increase of three pounds, about one pound is muscle and two pounds are fat. Very lean people, such as athletes, may gain even more muscle, and less fat. For example, Clark says she counseled a scrawny runner who gained 18 pounds during a year—17 of which were muscle. Recovering anorexics also rebuild lots of wasted muscle when they regain weight. They don't simply "get fat."

EASY COME, EASY GO?

Here's more good news from Clark: Weight that you gain quickly can be lost quickly provided you eat appropriately. Mother Nature will help you maintain a proper weight if you eat when you are hungry and stop when you are content—just like kids do.

In the twins study mentioned above, the overfed subjects lost 82 percent of the gained weight within four months through regular exercise and a prudent diet, while the twins with a family history of obesity kept more of the weight than those from leaner families.

GOING FOR THE BURN

Want to get rid of the evidence fast? Exercise will help keep the home fires (your metabolism) burning, so instead of sitting on the couch and groaning, "Oh, noooooo, I ate too much," take a nice, long walk or hop on your bicycle and go for a ride.

This isn't going to work miracles, mind you. You'd have to run a mile to burn off two excess Oreos, bike 30 minutes to burn off that extra muffin, and as for the piece of pie, the penance is 30 to 35 minutes of speedwalking.

In fact—and Clark says people are always shocked to learn this—exercise accounts for only a small proportion of the average person's daily calorie expenditure. Most of what you eat is used just to maintain your body, or your resting metabolic rate. To figure out how many calories you need just to exist, calculate your resting metabolism by simply multiplying your current weight (or appropriate weight, if you are significantly overweight) by 10 calories per pound.

For example, if you weigh 120 pounds, you need about 1,200 calories (10 × 120) simply to breathe, pump blood, and exist. Your brain, heart, kidneys, and liver represent only 5–7 percent of your weight, but contribute about 67 percent of the resting metabolic rate. In contrast, muscles represent about 40 percent of body mass but contribute only 24–26 percent of resting metabolic needs. According to the *New England Journal of Medicine,* your muscles burn 24 percent, your liver 26 percent, your brain 20 percent, your kidneys 10 percent, and your spleen 4 percent. And believe it or not, even your body fat burns calories—or five percent.

A 120-pound person would have to walk about 13 miles to expend the same number of calories burned in 24 hours at rest! During a standard workout, you may burn an additional 200 to 500 calories, but this is much less than what you'd need to stay alive for a day.

EVERYDAY CALORIES YOU NEED

Injured athletes or people taking a rest day from exercise sometimes forget that they need to eat despite the fact that they're not exercising. They think they deserve to eat only if they have exercised. Not so!

Assuming you are moderately active during the day (apart from your purposeful exercise), figure you'll need about 600 calories for coming and going to work, grocery shopping, and other activities of daily living for a grand total of 1,800 calories.

Just because you eat a little more doesn't mean you're automatically going to blimp out. Your body needs calories just as a fire needs wood—about 1,800 calories, in fact, just to go about your daily business and maintain your weight. (Of course, if you're trying to lose weight, 1,200 to 1,500 calories may be more appropriate, but never less than that.)

So don't let an occasional eating spree get you down. Mother Nature will handle the excess just fine—and given the natural limitations of your digestive tract, you probably won't be able to overeat enough at one sitting to gain more than a temporary pound or two.

To reiterate: To gain one little pound, you have to eat an additional 3,500 calories. That would be like wolfing down a huge Christmas day dinner—a heaping plate of turkey, mashed potatoes and gravy, stuffing, rolls and butter, eggnog, and a slice of apple pie and pecan pie à la mode and a few pieces of fudge, then in a few hours, doing it all over again the same day. Even I can't eat that much! In fact, even Beaver can't, and he's a REAL pig.

A QUESTION OF CHOLESTEROL

Since we're also going to be talking a lot about cholesterol in this book, let's go over a few basics. Once you understand what cholesterol is and what your cholesterol count is, you'll be better able to determine how much cholesterol and fat you can safely eat.

What is cholesterol? It's a type of fat found in all animals (including humans) and animal foods, including red meat, poultry, fish, and dairy products.

There are two types of cholesterol: HDL, or high-density lipoproteins—"good" cholesterol, because it carries the bad cholesterol out of the arteries—and LDL, low-density cholesterol, or "bad" cholesterol. This waxy substance contributes to hardening of the arteries and accumulates on the walls of the blood vessels throughout the body, especially in the heart. This buildup limits blood flow to the heart muscle and contributes to heart attacks.

Your Cholesterol Count

You can get your cholesterol level checked at any doctor's office with a simple blood test. In fact, many shopping malls and health fairs offer free cholesterol testing. As with body types and fat pockets, you may inherit a tendency for a high or low cholesterol count. If your family has a history of heart trouble, don't wait another page to cut the fat from your diet.

Recently, doctors have established that a cholesterol level of over 240 puts you at risk for heart attack and stroke; some doctors believe the risk begins at 200. Studies show the majority of heart attacks occur in individuals with cholesterol levels over 200. The higher the HDL percentage, the lower the risk of heart problems. At least 25 percent of your total blood cholesterol should be HDL.

If you divide your total cholesterol by your HDL level, your ratio should be about three to one. If your total is 200 and your HDL is 100, on the other hand, you're probably much healthier. A cholesterol level of 160 and an HDL of 105 is an excellent balance.

Your medical background also factors in, however. For instance, if your blood cholesterol level is less than 180 and you come from healthy stock (your grandparents are in their nineties and still kicking, maybe running marathons), you may be able to eat a little more fat than someone whose family background indicates a tendency toward heart disease.

Cholesterol in Food

The best way to keep your cholesterol count low is to avoid foods high in fat, especially saturated animal fat found in fatty hamburgers, pepperoni, hot dogs, sausage, whole dairy products, butter and lard. Replace them with low-fat foods such as grains, vegetables, and fish. Also, replace saturated oils with polyunsaturated or monounsaturated oils like canola oil, olive oil, safflower, or sunflower oils, suggests Hoxter.

By consuming 20 to no more than 30 percent* calories from fat per day and exercising regularly, you should never have a problem keeping your cholesterol count low. In fact, because exercise usually boosts HDL, that's one more excellent reason to become active on a regular basis (see Chapters 6–9 for more details on exercise programs).

---

*Thirty percent is the upper limit set by national organizations; we recommend aiming for the low twenties.

GETTING MOTIVATED

When I was 22 years old, I had a life-threatening blood clot and had to be hospitalized for six weeks. I was scared to death! But after the fear of amputation passed, I spent the next two months relearning how to walk and debunking the analysis from my doctor that I'd never be able to compete again. Well, not only did I overcome that frightening obstacle, I also went on to win six Ms. Olympia championships. So when it comes to motivation, inspiration, and energy, I speak from personal experience.

PATIENCE MAKES PERFECT

First things first: Don't expect overnight miracles. If you work hard and consistently, your efforts will blossom over a period of time, so don't expect to change years of bad eating and lack of exercise overnight. Just as it takes time to get out of shape, it takes time to get into shape.

Patience is something I have learned through years of painting. For instance, I can spend hours painting one eye. Each stroke brings me one step closer to the final product. But it's the sum of all the strokes that ultimately creates the masterpiece full of feeling and emotion.

The same principle applies to your body and physical fitness. If you expect overnight results, you're setting yourself up for disappointment. When I was training for Ms. Olympia, there were times when I would get frustrated because I was working so hard yet wasn't in the shape I wanted to be in. Then, the last two weeks before competition, everything always seemed to fall into place. But it wasn't my workouts in those last two weeks that got me there. It was the sum of all my workouts put together.

Whenever I get impatient and want to see results faster, I think of my body as a work of art. Each workout is like the stroke of a paint brush bringing me one step closer to my desired results.

Work hard and be consistent, and you can except change in direct proportion to your time and effort.

HOW TO GET AND STAY ON A ROLL

Have you ever tried to start riding a bike on a slight incline? It's pretty hard to get going from a stopped position, isn't it? It's the same with an exercise program. As Newton put it, bodies in motion tend to stay in motion—and that includes you.

When I haven't painted for a while, it always takes me so much time to get started. What do I want to paint? What size? Do I have the right tools? But once I get rolling, I'm fine. The more I paint and the more results I see, the more motivated I am to keep moving.

Exercise is the same. The hardest part about getting in shape is getting yourself started. The more you procrastinate, the less energy you have. And let's face it—coming up with all those excuses can really wear a girl out! Once you start exercising and eating right, you've smashed the inertia and are on a roll—hopefully a permanent one. (Like for the rest of your life!)

Beat at the end of the day and too pooped even to turn on the tube? All the more reason to exercise. Thirty minutes and you'll be so energized you'll feel as if you just woke up and ate a bowl of Wheaties.

So don't procrastinate, don't resist, and don't be afraid of the perceived costs of success or you'll remain stuck and stationary. Just jump in. Once you gain momentum, you're halfway there.

GAINING THE UPPER HAND

Much of how we control our attitudes, moods, and feelings comes from how we feel about ourselves. Life can be a roller coaster if you let it—up, down, up, down—pretty scary and unpredictable.

Positive people who feel good about themselves can often turn a negative situation into a positive one, or at least survive the experience without being devastated. The key is to gain control from the inside out.

What does that really mean? Accepting yourself, for starters—and getting in shape is the first step. It will change the way you feel about yourself as well as your mental outlook on everything happening around you. Suddenly you're glowing—it's like a contagious energy—something you wish you could bottle and share with others.

Those who dwell on negatives or failure are often fearful and lacking in confidence. This not only erodes your sense of control but chisels away at your inner sense of worthiness, resulting in low self-esteem. So be positive, realistic—and go for it!

LET GO OF GUILT

Nobody's perfect—not even those fashion models on magazine covers. (Ever heard of airbrushing? It not only can remove wrinkles but sometimes lots of pounds as well.)

If you've ever missed a workout, pigged out, or caught yourself acting like a couch potato, you know how powerful the guilt can be. You didn't live up to your expectations and you feel you've let yourself down.

Guilt can become psychological suicide that can inhibit your actions and destroy your self-confidence and self-respect. Ultimately, it is as destructive psychologically as cancer is physically. Like a rolling stone that gathers moss, guilt gets bigger and bigger until you feel negative not just about the "bad" thing you did, but yourself in general. Talk about making a mountain out of a molehill!

People have different ways of dealing with guilt. Some get stuck and can't move; others go into a blind frenzy and exercise until they're ready to drop, but they feel angry the entire time. Both extremes are unhealthy. Before succumbing to guilt, ask yourself where it's getting you. Is there anything redeeming about the guilt, or is it just a colossal waste of your time and energy?

Remember that you are human and there is always room for error. Missing a workout is not the end of the world. Learn to laugh at your defeats and use them as learning experiences. Reframe the negative into a positive. Meanwhile, console yourself with these three workout facts:

1. Accomplishing 15 percent of a workout is better than doing nothing at all. Can't bear the thought of speedwalking a half hour? Do 10 minutes (and I'll bet you get so energized you do the whole thing anyhow!)
2. Don't wait for things to be perfect to start. You may wait the rest of your life. For instance, "Oh, I'll start this workout after I answer all my calls, or after I do the dishes."
3. Set realistic goals. Don't expect perfection—just the best you can realistically be. Make that your goal—not some magazine cover.

HOW TO SET GOALS

I have a room in my house that Beaver, my pet pig, used to live in—until he got too big and I had to move him outside to his own little house. Meanwhile, I wanted him to feel comfortable in his room—like he was among friends. So I decided to paint a jungle scene on his walls.

Before I so much as picked up a paint brush, I painted a mental picture of what I wanted it to look like. The animals had to be friendly, and each had to have enough space to roam. I planned which animals would go on which walls—the lions and elephants could rest calmly on the large wall, the giraffes could gallop away in the distances, and the monkeys could hang out in the branches.

You wouldn't believe (in fact I still don't quite believe it myself) how easy it was to paint his room. Before I knew it, it was a jungle in there. And Beaver? He was one happy camper with all his friends around.

The room was a cinch to paint because I had a specific goal in mind, which was to make Beaver more comfortable, and it was something I was excited to do, which kept me motivated.

Reaching your fitness goals happens in the same way. You have to create a clear mental picture of what you want to achieve. Close your eyes for a second and visualize yourself in peak shape, then envision doing physical activities you really love. Finally, what have you always dreamed of doing that getting in great shape would finally let you do? Here are Seven Rules that can help you turn goals into reality.

In addition, you may want to go one step further and read the motivating self help books by authors Stephen R. Covey, Wayne W. Dyer, David J. Schwartz, Denis Waitley or Napoleon Hill.

SEVEN RULES FOR REAL FITNESS

1. Set Goals with a Reason in Mind

Your ultimate goal is happiness, right? Let's say you want to lose 10 pounds. Ask yourself why. Because my clothes will fit better? Because I'll look better and feel better about myself? Because I'll be healthier and live longer? Maybe your reasons are one or all of the above. Know what they are before you get started and your motivation will automatically build.

Would you start a long car drive without knowing your destination? Of course not. Set goals that are backed by your own strong desire.

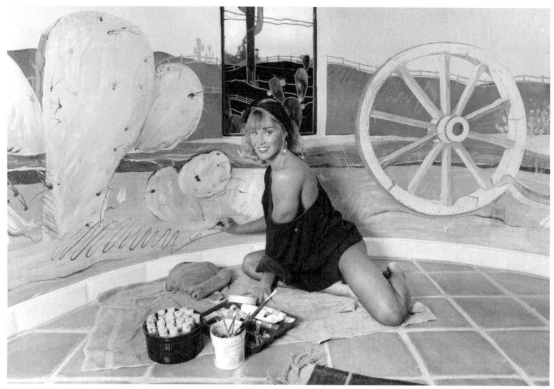

Creating a mental picture of what you want is an important first step in your fitness program. I always plan ahead—whether I'm painting a room or doing pushups.

2. Do it for Yourself!

Not your boyfriend, mother-in-law, distant cousin, or Santa Claus. YOU. While advice from family and friends is fine, if you don't really want it, their advice will sound like nagging—and we all know what we do when someone nags us. Nothing!

3. Accept Responsibility for Achieving Your Goal

Go ahead, own it. It's yours, so set up a game plan and get moving. Take that first step and you'll put yourself in the right mind-set to achieve your goal. Remember—think positive: You're a winner. Go for your goal 100 percent. It's all about trying, so don't give up!

4. Give Yourself a Concrete but Realistic Deadline

Let's face it. If we had forever to get in shape, it would probably take us that long. But we don't have forever; we only have now. Setting a deadline will work like a little kick in the pants to jump-start you into action. By creating in a sense of urgency, due dates can help prevent you from coming up with endless excuses. And if you're anything like me, you probably have a million of them ready to rip.

If your ultimate goal is to lose 50 pounds, break it up into minigoals with minideadlines.

For instance, plan to lose two pounds the first week and eight pounds by the end of the first month—a safe and realistic goal, which sounds a heck of a lot easier than losing all 50 at once.

Also, not only is it easier to foresee losing eight pounds at a time rather than 50 in one fell swoop, but you can reward yourself along the way and use the thrill of victory to keep losing more until you achieve your final goal. Achieving many small goals will fortify you for the long haul. It's like giving yourself a pat on the back to keep you motivated.

5. Develop a Plan of Attack

How do you plan to reach those goals and what steps will get you there? Also, what are you willing to put up with or do without to get there?

If you want to lose eight pounds, you must step up your activity and eat less or maybe change your eating patterns. If you're currently a couch potato, that means exercising 3 to 4 times a week for at least 20 minutes at a stretch. Figure out where you can carve out those hours from your week and plug them in. When I was an interior designer, my time for training was really crunched, so I simply got up a half hour early and worked out then and used my lunch hour for a workout. Did it work? You bet! I won national competitions that year. Decide what steps are necessary to reach your goals. Then, figure out how you're going to follow through.

6. Get It Down on Paper

It's essential to write your goals down. That way, they're permanent and there's no chance of fudging them. The list can also be a great visual tool. Try writing your goals in two-foot letters, cut from newspaper, and hang them somewhere you'll see them everyday. Or stick reminders on your bathroom mirror or on the fridge. If you really want your goals to be embedded in your memory for life, mimic those old schoolteachers and force yourself to write it down over and over and over—until you could write it in your sleep.

7. Leave Room for Obstacles and Opportunities

Life usually doesn't flow in a straight line, so don't set yourself up for a foolproof journey from fat to fit (or whatever your particular starting point happens to be).

Anticipate detours, obstacles—even total screwups and pig outs—but don't let them bum you out or derail you. Just look at them as inevitable potholes on the route to fitness and pick yourself up, dust yourself off, and press on!

For example, I suffered a shoulder injury while training for a Ms. Olympia competition. I could have given up and not entered that year, but I had been working toward that goal for months and hated to throw it all down the toilet. So rather than changing my goal, I changed the direction of my workout program to focus on a different body part—and around the injury—concentrating on my legs until I could use my arms again. Guess what happened? That year, I was known for having the best legs on stage—and won!

The pessimist sees the half glass of water as half empty, the optimist, as half full. It's still the same old half-glass of water. The only difference is how you perceive it. So embrace those detours, because who knows? Sometimes detours lead you to less obvious solutions that you never would have discovered had you stuck to the main drag.

SUMMING UP

Okay, ladies, start your engines. Put aside your fear, because fear leads to failure, and besides, once you get started you'll be too busy and happy to feel fear—and too motivated to stop. Don't waste your energy dreaming up excuses. Instead, dream up goals, visualize what you really want to look like, write or draw your goals in three-foot letters. And most of all—keep the faith. Think winner, not loser. Happiness, not sadness; fit, not fat. Make your fitness program a game that's fun, exciting, and challenging. As Descartes once said: I think, therefore I am. Think of yourself as becoming fit and healthy and before you know it, you will be! Don't look back, complain, or feel sorry for yourself. Be thankful for what you do have and never take that for granted.

In Chapter 2, we'll show you some ways to determine if you're overweight or just a "fat head," and how to combine a healthful, low-fat eating and exercise program for permanent and foolproof weight loss.

FEAR OF FAT

Fortunately, many women, having educated themselves in the school of sensible eating and exercise habits, are bucking the model-thin image that has pervaded for so long. In the realization that only a small percentage of women have the genetic makeup to look like fashion models without starving themselves, many women have settled on a weight that is comfortably healthy for them.

Morton G. Harmatz, Ph.D., a psychology professor at the University of Massachusetts in Amherst, conducted studies on women who "feel" fat but technically are normal or even underweight.

These women tended to punish and deprive themselves to lose imaginary excess weight. In addition to feeling fat, they generally had poor self-esteem, were more depressed, and were obsessed with weight loss efforts—often to the exclusion of other activities.

By contrast, overweight women in his study were far less likely to misperceive their weight and usually accurately defined themselves as overweight.

In fact, three-fourths of the underweight women considered themselves to be normal weight while a third of the normal weight women thought they were overweight. Only two percent of the overweight subjects thought they were normal weight. In other words, underweight women had a more distorted body image than those who were normal or overweight.

Women with distorted body images also suffered the following problems:

- They were far more preoccupied with weight and dieting and experienced more frustration and self-consciousness than those in the control group.
- They tended to diet continuously—whether they needed to or not, and expressed guilt and regret after eating certain foods, in particular, carbohydrates.
- They liked themselves better when they were dieting.
- They admitted that they used food to fill emotional voids—eating not because they were hungry but because they felt upset, angry, frustrated, or bored.
- They were more likely to daydream about food or to engage in mindless eating while watching television, talking on the phone, etc.
- Many resorted to fasting, appetite suppressants, and weight loss "medications."

- Few viewed food as healthful fuel. Instead, food was the foe that made them fat.
- They assumed that others found them unattractive because they were "fat."
- They were terrified of becoming fatter.
- They relished the feeling of an empty stomach.
- They were far more likely to have eating disorders, such as binging and purging, and/or laxative abuse than the control group,
- Many blamed themselves for their imagined "fatness" and felt less valued by society.
- They considered weight loss and thinness top priorities in life.

If any of these sound familiar to you—and your friends and family look at you as if you're crazy when you complain that you're overweight—you may be suffering from a bad body image.

Even if you're technically overweight or even obese, dwelling on your weight problem is counterproductive and usually leads to obsessive, crash dieting. And as we've explained earlier, the only thing diets do is make you fatter.

Let's be honest with each other. We've all experienced several of the insecurities listed above. Whether they were born out of unrealistic societal pressures or our own imaginations doesn't matter. We need to admit, acknowledge, confront, and finally resolve them to move on to health—and away from dieting. We'll give you more advice on how to do that throughout this book, so keep reading! Even if you're 20 or more pounds overweight, don't despair. In this book, I'm going to teach you everything you need to know to uncover—once and for good—the beautiful body and person that's been hiding beneath that fat. We're in this together so just stick with me, and together we'll succeed. I promise . . . but give it a wholehearted chance!

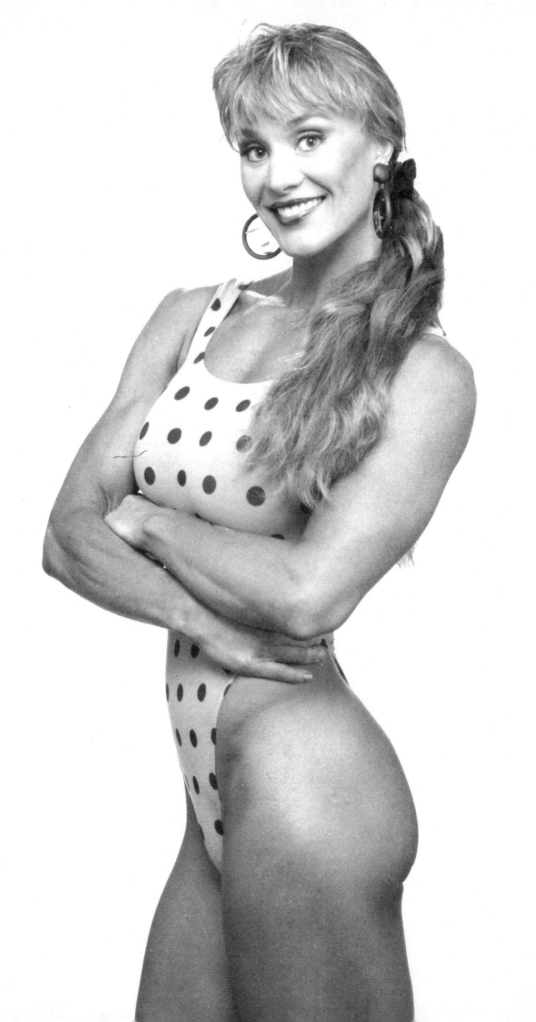

TWO

The Skinny on Fat

As we explained in the last chapter, many women think they're too fat—even if they're perfect for their size and frame. Blame it on years of "thinness" conditioning from the media and Hollywood, who have brainwashed us into believing that unless we're built like a model, we're flawed or maybe just too lazy or undisciplined to achieve "The Look." Now even models have exercise videos showing how they have to work their butts off—to keep their butts off.

Studies show that only five percent of women have the genetic makeup to achieve model-thinness. As for the rest of us, our ancestry has put limits on how tall, thin, even how shapely we can ever be.

I can almost hear what you're thinking. Well, alright. If I can't fix it myself, I'll go to a plastic surgeon and get it vacuumed out or chopped off. But that's often not a viable solution, either, as plastic surgeons as well as a few unsuspecting victims who went "under the knife" will share in the next chapter.

In fact, I have a few friends who underwent liposuction. For a few months following the procedure they looked great. But within six months they had regained all the weight and looked exactly as they had before. The only thing that was still slimmer was their wallets. Liposuction is not a permanent solution. It appears that Mother Nature has her own agenda for the "shape" women are naturally to assume. If she intended us all to have flat stomachs, perhaps we'd all have been born that way.

I don't mean to suggest you're stuck with thunder thighs or tummy bulge; just that a low-fat diet and regular exercise program are the only permanent ways to bring them in line.

NEW WAVE OF LOSING WEIGHT

As we explained at the end of Chapter 1, many women see fat when there isn't any there and use their fear as a cloak to avoid other issues in life.

While the bad news is that new research shows that one of every two women still believes that she's overweight (government health statistics says only one-quarter actually are), the good

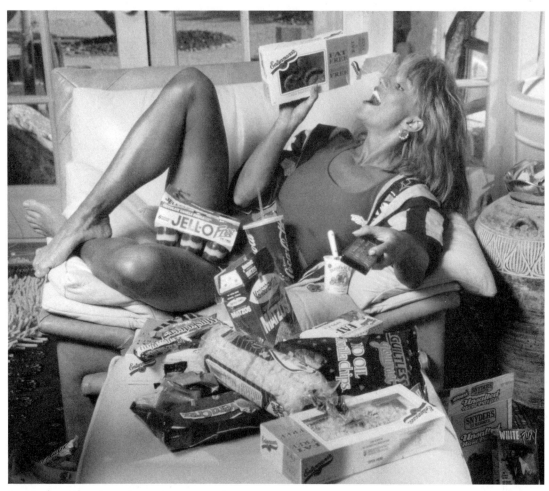

Let the new line of non-fat cookies, cakes, and other goodies help you hold the line on flab. Non-fat options allow you to have your cake and eat it too.

news is that at least we're resorting to far healthier ways to lose this imaginary excess weight. The trend is away from old-fashioned dieting à la starvation, calorie counting, and diet pills, toward using low-fat and low-calorie foods to lose weight, says John Foreyt, Ph.D., professor at Baylor College of Medicine, who has studied the psychology of weight control for 25 years.

A study conducted by the Calorie Control Council showed that 88 percent of those who consider themselves overweight are consuming either low-calorie or reduced-fat beverages to lose weight, while only 47 percent of these people say they're on a "diet." It just becomes part of their lifestyle. After all, it's as easy to grab the fat-free salad dressing as the fat-filled version next to it, right?

Helping the trend along is a boom in non- and low-fat versions of the real thing. If you've checked your grocery shelves lately, you'll see these products are virtually crowding the fatty stuff off the shelves.

In fact, about 520 new low-fat/low-cholesterol foods were introduced in seven food categories in 1992—a 39 percent increase over 1991. FIND/SVP, a market research firm, says that by the year 2000, every type of food sold in retail and food service outlets will be available in a low-fat or low-cholesterol alternative. I'm putting in my bid for non-fat chocolate cheese cake. Talk about something to look forward to!

Today, the most popular ways to lose weight, according to the Calorie Control Council's 1993 survey, are:

- Cutting down on high-calorie, high-fat foods, (98 percent)
- Using low-fat foods and beverages (92 percent)
- Exercise (90 percent)
- Low-calorie foods and beverages (85 percent)

Losing favor among weight-losers are:

- Counting calories (39 percent)
- Skipping meals (21 percent)
- Diet substitutes (17 percent)
- Diet pills (3 percent)

A MATTER OF GENES

But back to my original question. Are you really too fat for your size and frame? And how can you tell for sure? Most of us know. I mentioned earlier that when my cheeks (upper and lower sets) get plump and make me look like a chipmunk with a fat rump, it's off to the gym I go (and away with the Snickers bars) regardless of how thin my boyfriend claims I look.

According to Wayne Calloway, M.D., an endocrinologist and director of the Center for Clinical Nutrition at George Washington University Medical Center (he's conducted studies of obese women for more than 20 years), if you find it impossible to lose weight it could be because you're simply not meant to be any thinner. You could be battling a series of messages encoded in your genes. But even if you can't be modern-thin—and remember, most of us can't, no matter how hard we try—you can be a firmer and more shapely version of you.

Eighty percent of the variations of body weight is genetically determined—just like the color of your eyes or the shape of your nose. Scientists at many obesity clinics, including Rockefeller University in New York, report that obese patients lose dozens of pounds, go home, and come back six months later having regained exactly the amount they lost—to the half pound.

By the same token, the body also resists major weight gain—no doubt a comforting thought to some of you. In a classic study conducted in the 1960s at the University of Vermont, a group of 20 prisoners of normal weight volunteered to gain as much weight as possible. Only by forcing themselves to dramatically overeat by thousands of calories a day did they manage to gain 20 pounds. When the study ended, they all returned to their normal weight.

While researchers don't understand why the body seems to have a narrow weight range, they believe it may be linked to some sort of biochemical control system. We're not saying that your genetically programmed weight is necessarily a healthy one—especially if you're genetically programmed toward obesity. But it may not be the result of a piggish appetite, either.

DIETING DOOM

The other major cause of weight gain, of course, is dieting. Call it a case of rapidly shrinking metabolism, but the more you diet, the more your metabolism slows down until it becomes increasingly difficult to lose unwanted pounds. If you lose 20 pounds, 15 of them are fat and the other five are muscle. But when you regain weight, you regain 18 pounds of fat and only two pounds of muscle. Who ever said life was fair?

"Unless you're morbidly obese, eating less than 10 calories per pound of body weight daily could sabotage your weight loss efforts by signaling your body to resist your every attempt to reduce. You'd lose more on a sensible 1,400 calorie diet than by starving yourself on 800 calories," says Calloway.

BAD MATH—NOT METABOLISM

Finally, another reason people fail at weight loss is because they underestimate how much they really eat. A study conducted at St. Luke's Roosevelt Hospital in New York, which analyzed the self-reported calorie intake and expenditures of people who claimed they had problems losing weight, showed that the "diet-resistant" group consumed about twice as many calories as reported and exercised one-fourth less. Apparently it was their faulty math—not their metabolism—that was making it hard for them to lose weight. (Or maybe their minds were swaying their sense of reality to alleviate guilt?) If you fall into this group, here's a few devices that can help you keep track of the evidence:

- *Bowe's and Church's Food Values of Portions Commonly Used,* 14th Edition, revised by Jean A.T. Pennington (Lippincott, 1984)
- *Health Counts: A Fat and Calorie Guide,* by Kaiser Permanente (Wiley, 1991)
- *Fast Food Facts: Nutrition and Exchange Values for Fast-Food Restaurants,* by Marion J. Franz, third edition (DCI Publishers, 1990)
- *The International Cuisines Calorie Counter,* by Denise Webb (M. Evans, 1990)

It also helps to know how many calories you really burn through exercise and physical activities. We'll cover this more thoroughly in Chapters 6–9, but here's a chart to help you determine if you're burning as many calories as you think you are during exercise.

Jogging (6 mph): About 580–750 calories per hour
Slow walking (2.5 mph): About 200–250 calories per hour
Brisk walking (4 mph): About 250–350 calories per hour
Aerobic dance: About 480–650 calories per hour
Cycling (9 mph): About 300–500 calories per hour
Tennis (singles): About 315–480 calories per hour

BIG THREE QUESTIONS

Okay, let's shake off some pounds here, ladies. To find a weight-loss program that works, ask yourself three questions.

1. Do I really need to lose weight?
2. How much do I need to lose?
3. What is the safest, most effective way to lose it permanently?

WHO SHOULD LOSE WEIGHT?

Today, about 20 percent of the American population is 20 percent overweight. If you suffer from medical complications because you're overweight, such as diabetes, high blood pressure, and a high percentage of body fat (more than 35 percent for women and we'll show you how to determine yours in a minute), you may be a good candidate for weight loss. Hypertension develops ten times more often in women who are 20 percent or more overweight, and diabetes occurs three times more often among obese people. By losing just 20 percent of their excess weight, obese women can reduce coronary heart disease risks by 40 percent–not a bad investment for your time, when you think of it.

SO DO YOU REALLY NEED TO LOSE WEIGHT?

You're probably at your ideal weight or very close to it if:

- Your waist to hip ratio (WHR) is less than .80 (See p. 41 to calculate.)
- Your blood cholesterol is less than 200 milligrams per decimeter
- Your HDL (high density lipoprotein cholesterol count) is 45 or lower
- Your family has no history of heart disease or diabetes
- You have normal blood pressure
- You engage in at least 30 minutes of aerobic exercise three times weekly
- You eat a high-fiber, low-fat diet with no more than 30 percent calories from fat

On the other hand, if the following list describes you better, it's time to use this program to shed some excess pounds.

- Your BMI (Body Mass Index) is higher than 25
- Your waist-to-hip (WHR) ratio is higher than .80 (see p. 41)
- Your blood cholesterol is higher than 200 mg/dl
- Your HDL is less than 35
- You are sedentary

- You consume a high-fat diet (lots of red meat, dairy products, junk foods)
- You smoke
- You drink a lot of alcohol
- You have high blood pressure
- Your family has a history of heart disease or adult-onset diabetes

WHY MODELS SHOULD NOT BE YOUR MODELS

Before we show you how to determine if you're overweight, we'd like to ask you a big favor. Put away those fashion magazines! Models are generally not models of health. In fact, Simonson explains that many are dangerously underweight and resort to unhealthful dietary practices to remain that way.

For decades the prevailing definition of what a woman's shape should look like has caused an increase in eating problems and tremendous pressure on women to starve themselves into a shape they were never meant to be. Twenty years ago, professional models and Miss America contestants were about five to 10 percent below the average weight for their height. Today, it's even worse: the typical model peering at you from the pages of *Elle, Vogue,* or *Mademoiselle* is 20 to 25 percent below her average weight. That means she weighs just three-fourths of what is healthy for her, explains Simonson.

In January, 1992, *People* magazine interviewed three top models—Kim Alexis, Carol Alt, and Beverly Johnson—for their cover story. All three admitted that they had frequently resorted to binging, purging, and fasting to retain their svelte, cover-girl physiques. While all three have since adopted more healthful eating and exercise programs, it was a long and hard uphill struggle to regain their health—and one that is paved with temptations to slip back into old routines. (See Chapter 10 for more details on how the industry puts pressure on models to diet down to unrealistic weights.)

Are you really overweight or just feeling fat, as we discussed in Chapter 1? My tried-and-true detection method is to simply look in the mirror or try on my favorite jeans. Of course, there are far more scientific options to use if you prefer. Here are a few.

Measure the Evidence

At what point is too much fat dangerous to your health? Scientists use a measure called the body mass index, or BMI, which incorporates both height and weight. You can find your own BMI by following these simple instructions.

To measure your BMI:

1. Multiply your weight in pounds by 700.
2. Divide by your height in inches.
3. Divide by your height again. Your BMI is the end result.

Scientists consider a BMI below 25 most healthful, while 25–30 is considered moderately overweight and carries a slight risk of weight-related problems such as high blood pressure, blood cholesterol, heart disease, and Type 11 diabetes (non-insulin dependent).

If your score is higher than 30, you're at high risk—which means it's time to cut the fat.

Studies show that people with a lifelong BMI of less than 25 percent have the lowest rate of heart disease, premature death, cancer, and cardiovascular disease.

Another way to measure your fat content is the waist-to-hip ratio, or WHR. This ratio distinguishes between apples, or people (usually men) who carry their weight above the waist, and pears (usually women) who carry their excess weight around the hips and buttocks.

To measure your WHR:

1. Place a measure tape at the narrowest point in your waist with your stomach relaxed. Waist in inches =
2. Measure the circumference of your hips at their widest point, or where your buttocks protrude the most. Hips in inches =
3. Divide your waist measurement by your hip measurement: Waist/hip = waist-to-hip ratio.

If your waist is more than 80 percent of the circumference of your hips, you should lose some weight. The higher above 80 percent the waist/hip ratio, the greater your health risk. In fact, scientists now believe that WHR may be a better predictor of fat-related diseases than weight.

In the future, CAT scans and other, more sophisticated tests may be able to differentiate between different types of fat. Meanwhile, a big belly may be your best guide. If you can't see the floor and you're not seven months pregnant, it's time to act. In fact, a pot or beer belly— even on an otherwise very thin woman—could signal serious health problems. See your physician immediately.

Excess abdominal fat is more dangerous than below-the-belt flab because it is associated with increased insulin resistance, which is a precursor to diabetes and may help cause hypertension. Interestingly, the risks of being overweight seem to diminish as we age, although scientists aren't sure why.

WEIGHING IN THE REAL WAY

And then there are all those weight-height charts. Will the real one please stand up? According to one, you're overweight; according to another, you're perfect; according to a third, you're underweight if you have a big frame (and you sure hope you do).

Probably the best chart around is the one put out by the Metropolitan Life Insurance Company, although you'll have to do some math to make sense of it because it measures height with one-inch heels and weight with three pounds of clothing. (Don't ask us why—we haven't figured it out, either.)

To determine whether your frame is small, medium, or large, look at your hands, wrists, and feet. If your wrist is thin and delicate and your feet are smaller than average for women your height, you may have a small frame. Conversely, if you have feet like flippers, you may have a large frame, although this is not a concrete rule.

Unless you weight train regularly and are really a buff, subtract three pounds from the maximum weight allowed. Muscle weighs more than fat, which is another reason to get fit. You have permission to weigh more!

Don't take the following chart as the gospel truth. It doesn't take into account how your weight is distributed or other important health factors. And why diet down to 135 pounds if you have to starve yourself to get and stay there? More important than what you weigh is how good you feel at a particular weight.

Height	Small	Medium	Large
4'10	102–111	109–121	118–131
4'11	103–113	111–123	120–134
5'1	106–118	115–129	125–140
5'2	108–121	118–132	128–143
5'3	111–124	121–135	131–147
5'4	114–127	124–128	134–151
5'5	117–130	127–141	137–156
5'6	120–133	130–144	140–159
5'7	123–136	136–150	143–163
5'8	126–139	136–150	146–167
5'9	129–142	139–153	149–170
6'0	138–151	148–162	158–179

Weighing yourself regularly is okay, provided you don't let a pound or two ruin your day, says Simonson. Some women, in fact, (and I'm not one of them), feel less anxious knowing exactly what they weigh than wondering and worrying if they've gained a pound or two. At least if you know the truth, you can do something about it. Wondering usually makes you worry more.

For others, a daily weigh-in makes or breaks the entire day. If the number is low, it's a good day. On the other hand . . . I have a friend who became so infuriated with her bathroom scale day after a week of starving and intense exercise that she heaved it out the window. Lest she be tempted to buy another, she framed the springs and hung them on her bathroom wall. It reminds her that while daily weigh-ins may be a boon for some, but for her it's a total bust.

However you weigh in, make sure you do so on a highly accurate bathroom scale—not one of those cheap floor models, which may vary by as much as five to seven pounds, depending on where you put them and how you stand on them. The truth is, I can get just about any weight I want to out of my inexpensive floor scale depending on where I place my feet and whether I put the scale on a hard floor or on a thick carpet, which "swallows" a few pounds. I sometimes weigh myself on a rug when I know I'm a little overweight; the lower number makes me feel better even though I know it's a lie. Sound familiar, anyone?

Remember that a scale measures far more than your actual weight. The grand total also includes muscle gains from your new weight-training program, that pizza you had for dinner, the two glasses of water you drank an hour ago, plus intestinal contents, clothing, shoes, and any jewelry you may be wearing.

Nancy Clark suggests that those who prefer a daily weigh-in do so at the same time of day—say, first thing in the morning after you've emptied your bladder.

If you weigh yourself after a vigorous workout, you may weigh five pounds less, but it's not a real weight loss, just water loss from sweat. Drink a few glasses of water and that "weight loss" will disappear before your very eyes.

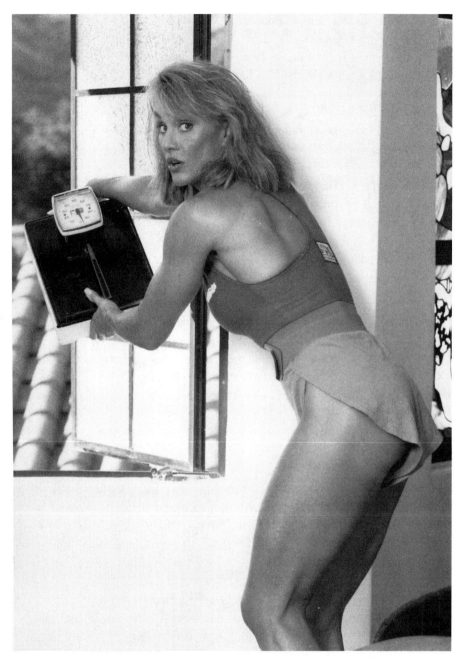

When the scale gives me the wrong number, I'm tempted to toss it out the window—as good an excuse as any for not weighing myself daily.

And whether you weigh yourself by the day, week, or month, remember that it's natural for weight to fluctuate by a pound or two. Also, nearly every woman "gains" a few extra pounds of "bloat" water weight in the days preceding her menstrual cycle. You know what I mean—those PMS days when your body feels like a stuffed sausage, and your brain seems waterlogged, too.

Finally, if you seem to gravitate toward a weight that is higher than your "ideal weight" by a pound or two, don't sweat it. Just try to learn to live with it. According to Simonson, studies show that carrying a little excess fat on your hips and thighs is more likely to hurt your vanity than your health.

MEASURING YOUR BODY FAT PERCENT

Your body-fat composition is the ratio of fat to lean body mass. In general, women whose body fat exceeds 30 percent are considered at a higher risk for chronic diseases such as diabetes, hypertension, and heart disease, while a body fat percentage below 12 percent, the case with many professional athletes and bodybuilders, may increase the risk of cessation or irregularity of menstruation, which can lead to bone thinning over a period of time if you don't increase fat intake.

Here's a rough estimate of what that percentage means to you:

- Below 10 percent: Dangerously low body fat
- Between 14 and 17 percent: Very low body fat
- 17 to 20: Healthfully low body fat
- 20 to 27: Average body fat
- 27 to 31: Unhealthfully high body fat
- Above 31: Dangerously high body fat.

Be forewarned that getting an accurate measurement isn't always easy, even when it's conducted by alleged "professionals." Some methods just aren't reliable, while other measurements can be thrown off by your intake of liquids, medications, and other factors. Nearly every health club and gym offers some sort of body fat testing, or you can do it yourself with less reliable results. If you're more than 20 pounds overweight, ask your physician to refer you to a specialist.

Skinfold Calipers

This is the easiest, fastest, most convenient, least expensive, and also the least accurate fat-testing method. In fact, a too-hasty measurement an inch above or below the established pinch zone (for women, it's usually at specific sites on the front of the thigh, the back of the upper arm, and the area over the hip bone; for men, the chest, abdomen, and thigh) can add 5 to 15 millimeters of fat to the measurement and translate into a falsely high reading. Individual patterns of fat distribution also may result in false readings. For instance, if you have heavy arms but an otherwise slender body, your arms will yield a false high reading.

Many health clubs use skinfold calipers. If the tester is experienced (not always the case), the results may be fairly accurate. For instance, you may measure 23 whereas you're actually 25 or 26 percent fat. However, it's far more accurate than someone simply looking at you and determining that you're too fat, which often results in a margin of error of 12 to 15 percent.

Different testers may select different sites to measure, so it's important to get the same instructor to retest you since she may be more likely to measure the same sites. Remember, however, that even with careful testing there are likely to be unavoidable discrepancies. For best results, make sure your tester was trained at the level of health-fitness instructor from the American College of Sports Medicine. Administering these tests requires skill as well as experience. Accuracy rate: C

Bioelectrical Impedance Tests

This is one of the newest body-fat testing methods around. Portable and relatively simple to use, it's become a popular addition to health fairs and athletic events. Unfortunately, it, too, has ac-

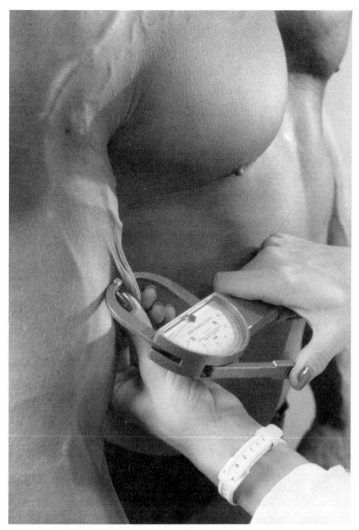

Skinfold calipers are the fastest way to "pinch" your body fat percentage. (It doesn't hurt!)

curacy problems. In this test, you lie on your back while an electrical signal is sent from an electrode on your foot to an electrode on your hand. The slower the signal travels, the more fat you have as compared to lean body mass, since fat carries relatively little water and water conducts electricity while fat impedes the signal.

But here's where problems come in: If you're dehydrated for any reason at all, that will throw off the test so you weigh "fatter" than you really are. A few situations that may cause an inaccurate reading include vigorous exercise just before the test, a bout with diarrhea, use of laxatives or diuretics, or consumption of dehydrating beverages with alcohol or caffeine. Hardcore athletes often get tested after a workout in the mistaken belief they'll measure lower. Fat chance!

On the other hand, if you're retaining water, have PMS, kidney problems, or you just drank a gallon of water, you may measure leaner.

Even if you're water-balanced and accurately positioned, you can still get an inaccurate reading because the test is based on the assumption that the standard person is 73 percent water. But young people tend to be 77 percent water and older people about 71 percent. The test can be very accurate if the tester is trained and you're neither dehydrated nor bloated.

With bioelectrical impedance testing, you receive a computer printout estimating your body-fat percentage and metabolic rate as well as suggested diets and exercise regimes. By choosing from the list of activities, the computer can tell you how many calories per minute you'll burn based on your current body weight. Accuracy Rate: B

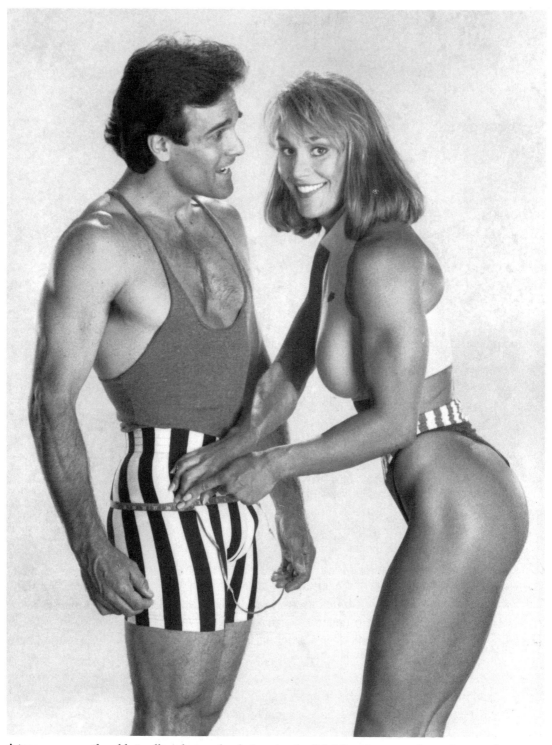

A tape measure, the old standby, also works—but again, don't let the wrong number ruin your day. Fluctuations—especially during PMS days—are normal.

Underwater Weighing

Underwater weighing is perhaps the most accurate testing mode; unfortunately, it is typically expensive and not widely available in more remote areas of the country. To undergo this test, you exhale all the air in your lungs and then are weighed while submerged in a tank of water. This technique doesn't measure body fat but body density, which is then translated into percentage fat.

Accuracy problems usually creep in during translation because the equations for translating density into fat have been determined for the "standard male," and women have a much different muscular build and bone density than men.

Errors are frequent because subjects get nervous and don't completely exhale all the air in their lungs before going underwater. Just two cups of air inside the body can affect body-fat measurement by as much as three to five percent. In fact, I remember when I did this. I was bobbing up and down because I couldn't blow all my air out.

Intestinal gas can also disrupt the accuracy, so be sure to avoid gas-producing foods before testing. Finally, substandard equipment is another culprit. Many of the portable underwater tanks used at health fairs and expos are not as precise as those used in research labs and may give false readings. Accuracy Rate: B+

Other Weighers and Measurers

Many spas and health clinics also have sophisticated computerized treadmills that measure your ideal weight with varying degrees of accuracy. Don't be awed by the bells and whistles—that $10,000 machine may be no more accurate than a $20 set of calipers.

Until researchers come up with a foolproof way to measure body fat, rather than taking it as the gospel truth, use your "score" as a comparison guide. No matter how they measure your fat, the standard error is about three percent plus or minus.

LISTEN TO YOUR BODY

Perhaps the best way to measure fat is to use your instincts, says Simonson. This is what I've always done—and it's absolutely free. I honestly believe that each of us has the ability to "know," as I do, when we are above or below the right fat percent and weight and that we can hone these instincts to a fine science.

Listen carefully to what your body tells you. If you're above your ideal weight, you may feel fat and flabby and your body will tell you to exercise more, and eat sparingly for a day or so to cleanse. If you're below your ideal fat percent, you may feel tense and jittery and your body may scream for carbohydrates or maybe just a break from training.

OTHER THINGS TO CONSIDER

Now that you have a few numbers to work with, let's consider other factors that figure into your ideal weight. Numbers are only part of the answer.

Fat cells are tiny reservoirs, and we're all born with a set number of them. While you can shrink them, you can't eliminate them completely. Try to remember how your weight was distributed when you were 18 years old. If weight or fat came on earlier in life, you will tend to have an increased number of fat cells and it will be harder for you to reduce your weight to match the standard weight tables.

Check your family tree. At your next family gathering, take stock of your immediate family and relatives. Are you shaped pretty much like everyone else? Everyone inherits a predisposition for having fat deposits at certain places on your body. For instance, if your mother has heavy calves and thin arms, you may well follow in her footsteps. Document your family history and look not only at your parents and siblings but also at your grandparents. Studies show obesity rarely occurs in people who have no family history of obesity. But people whose parents and grandparents were obese may be destined to be fat. Part of this may be due to eating habits that get passed down from one generation to the next—like recipes for pound cake. For instance, I inherited my mother's addiction for breads, coffee, and especially chocolate. Those darn German genes did it again. Thanks, Mom!

LOSERS ARE NOT ALL EQUAL

You've been weighed, measured, pinched, and dunked and the evidence is overwhelming: You need to lose some weight. Okay, first the bad news. There are several reasons why you might have a harder time losing weight than your best friend. These include a genetic disposition to being obese or overweight, a larger number of fat cells, and long-established habits of eating too much and not exercising enough.

But not to worry. In general, the right mix of proper diet, exercise, and behavioral and psychological intervention will enable you to shed those extra pounds—provided your weight-loss program fits you—not your best friend who may have a different genetic makeup or body shape.

THE SHAPE YOU'RE IN

Whether you like it or not, you've inherited a specific body type that you cannot completely change without drastic plastic surgery—and even that doesn't always work. Studies show that it's not only how much body fat you have but also where it's stored that influences how healthy you are and even how long you can expect to live. Your basic shape not only determines where you're likely to gain and lose weight, but may also increase your risks of developing particular conditions and diseases—but only if you're substantially overweight. If you're normal weight, the risks don't apply. Women (and men, too) tend to fall into three basic body categories:

1. Ectomorphs: Women with long legs and arms, narrow fingers and toes, and a delicate bone structure. Many long-distance runners, cyclists, and ballerinas are ectomorphs.
2. Mesomorphs: Women with a heavy bone and muscle development, broad hands, and a muscular chest. Gymnasts are often found in this group.
3. Endomorphs: Women who are round and soft, often with slender wrists and ankles and delicate facial features.

Within these three categories are two more subcategories, or what we call the fruit groups: Apples and Pears. Which are you? To find out, determine your waist to hip ratio (WHR). Grab a tape measure. Measure your waist at your naval, and your hips at their widest point. Now, divide the circumference of your hips by the circumference of your waist. If you're .80 or above, you're an apple. If you're below .80, you're a pear. (If you're horrible at math here's an easier way: If your waist is 36 inches or more, you're probably an apple.)

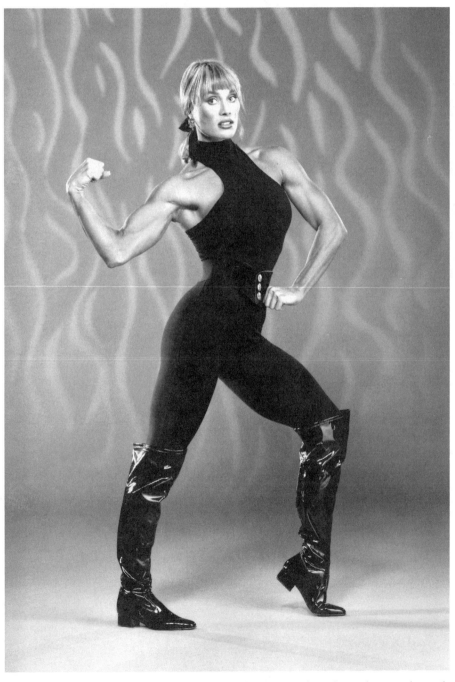

Mesomorphs, such as myself and most bodybuilders and gymnasts, have heavy bone and muscle development, broad hands, and a muscular chest.

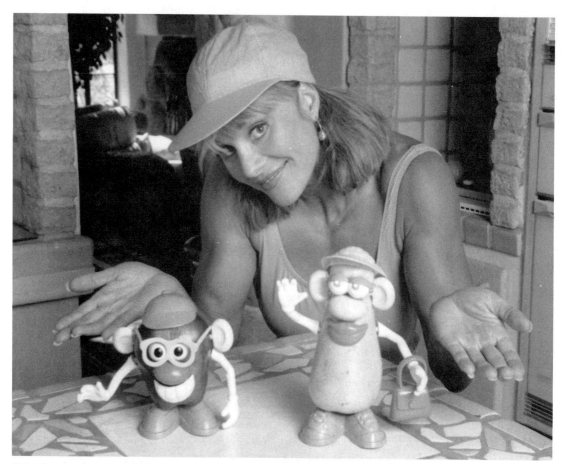

Whether you're an apple or a pear, you can reproportion your body with exercise.

APPLE-SHAPED WOMEN

Pick up an apple and take a close look at it. Notice how it's round in the middle and tapered at each end? If you're shaped roughly like that, with most of your extra weight in your chest and abdomen, you're an apple. Some apples store most of their fat near their internal organs, while others carry it close to their skin. (On the other hand, you might be like me: a Granny apple with naval orange tendencies—and a Chiquita banana/squash psychosis. Is there a doctor in the house?)

Most men are apple-shaped, especially as they approach middle age. Check out the over-35 bunch in your life to see what I mean. Even guys who were skinny as a rail in their twenties may have a slight paunch now. It's not necessarily their fault, or even the result of too many six-packs, but rather the male hormone, testosterone.

PEAR-SHAPED WOMEN

Now pick up a pear. Notice how most of the bulk of the fruit is about three-quarters of the way down? If you're a pear, most of your fat is below your belt in your hips and thighs, while the upper body is relatively slender. Most females tend to be pears. If your female friends are anything like mine, most of them complain about heavy hips and thighs—not beer bellies.

Is it possible to change your basic shape through a healthful weight-loss program of diet and exercise? Yes, but only if you're an apple. In other words, when an apple diets, she winds up looking more like a pear but a pear usually becomes a smaller pear.

THE TROUBLE WITH BIG APPLES

But we're talking more than fruit shapes here.

Elizabeth Somer, M.A., R.D., a registered dietitian and author of the *Nutrition Newsletter,* reported in *Shape* magazine that apples are more likely to develop a cluster of biological complications known as "metabolic syndrome." These changes are associated with a greater risk for heart disease, stroke, diabetes, high blood pressure, and gallbladder disease.

Research also shows that certain diseases linked to metabolic problems progress more rapidly in apples, and that apples often tend to die sooner than pears, even when both weigh the same and have similar body-fat percentages. Blood cholesterol and triglyceride levels also tend to be higher in apples while good cholesterol (HDL) is lower.

Overweight apples are also 15 times more likely to develop endometrial cancer, and five times more likely to develop breast cancer, than pear-shaped women. (Normal-weight apples are not at any greater risk than pears, however.) Studies show pot-bellied apples often suffer from overproduction of insulin, which can trigger high blood fat and blood glucose levels and that they have higher estrogen (or, for men, testosterone) levels which can increase their risks for certain cancers.

Don't crash diet! You'll wind up fatter, not thinner—and more prone to dangerous diseases like cancer and heart disease.

MEDIEVAL TO MODERN

We've come a long way from the voluptuous body that was popularized in the 1600s by great European artists. Just for fun and to provide a little perspective, let's take a quick look at how the "ideal" female body has changed down through the ages.

The "eternally pregnant woman," popularized in the 1600s by artists such as Michelangelo, was the voluptuous, reproductive, or maternal prototype, with a swelling, almost pregnant-like, belly, huge breasts, and a tiny waist. The buxom, voluptuous figure was not only considered fashionable but a healthful protection against starvation, disease, and famine. In fact, by the mid-1800s, physicians proclaimed extreme plumpness was a measure of physical as well as mental health.

From the late 1800s to World War I, the Gibson girl was the rage. Taller and thinner than her voluptuous predecessor, she retained a full bosom and hips. The combination introduced, for the first time in history since Cave Woman Jane ducked the club, the notion of the athletic-looking woman.

In the early 1900s, the Flapper danced on the scene with her boyish, slender figure. The women's movement had begun! The Flapper's thinness represented emancipation from traditional women's roles as childbearer and wife.

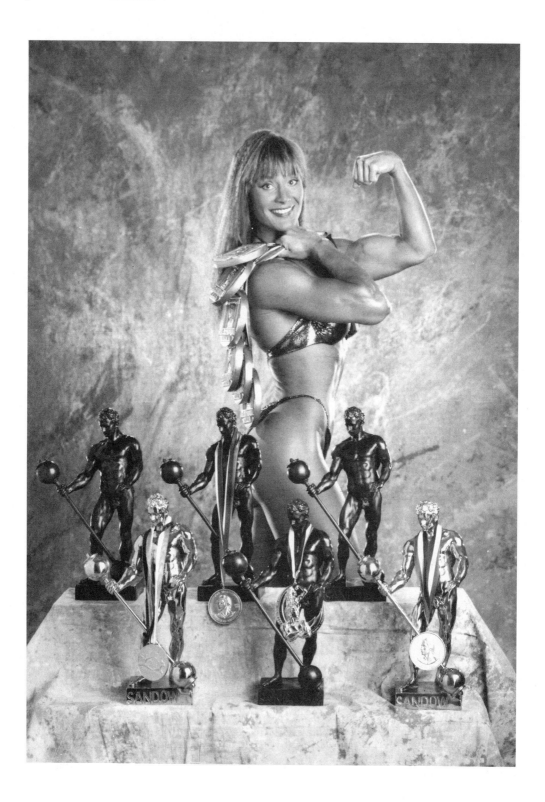

Ultra-thinness continued into the 1960s as models like Jean Shrimpton, Cheryl Tiegs, and Twiggy illustrated that women were moving away from traditional roles and into the workplace. The androgynous, fashion-model body became a symbol of equality between the sexes, especially in the workplace where women were starting to make substantial inroads.

Muscles on a woman were considered masculine as recently as 10 years ago. The only women around with biceps were professional bodybuilders and circus acrobats.

Then things began changing. A lot of slight, underdeveloped women—you know, the Sweet Pea types—suddenly began asking me how they could become stronger; barbells started appearing in women's gyms, and within a few years weight training was no longer considered weird but a normal and essential part of a healthful exercise program.

Jane Fonda was among the first to popularize muscles. Critics joked that the trend would pass, but by the mid-1980s, fashion magazines were proclaiming the new goal was not thinness but fitness. Suddenly, being in shape was chic, and muscles were not only okay but sexy. Everyone from Madonna to corporate executives was pumping iron.

Today, we're fortunate to live in a time when the "ideal" body just happens to be a most healthful one, or the body that best accommodates your genetic code and body frame. Although some fashion magazines continue to portray the ideal woman's body as pencil-thin, far more today are showing models with curves and even muscles. After all these years, we finally have cover girls who are healthful-looking, realistic role models. They don't have perfect bodies, either size or shape wise, but "real" bodies—which makes them all the more beautiful. Just ask any guy. He'll tell you.

The best advice I can give you is to make the most of the body you have. Focus on the parts of your body you like, not those you loathe. And concentrate on achieving better health rather than some predetermined "ideal" weight set forth by the insurance companies. Be realistic about how much you can really change about your body, and remember that female hormones supply natural padding in the hips and thighs. Finally, accept your body, thunder thighs and all. Less than 100 years ago, you would have been considered a great work of art. With this program, you can take that art and sculpt it into your own masterpiece.

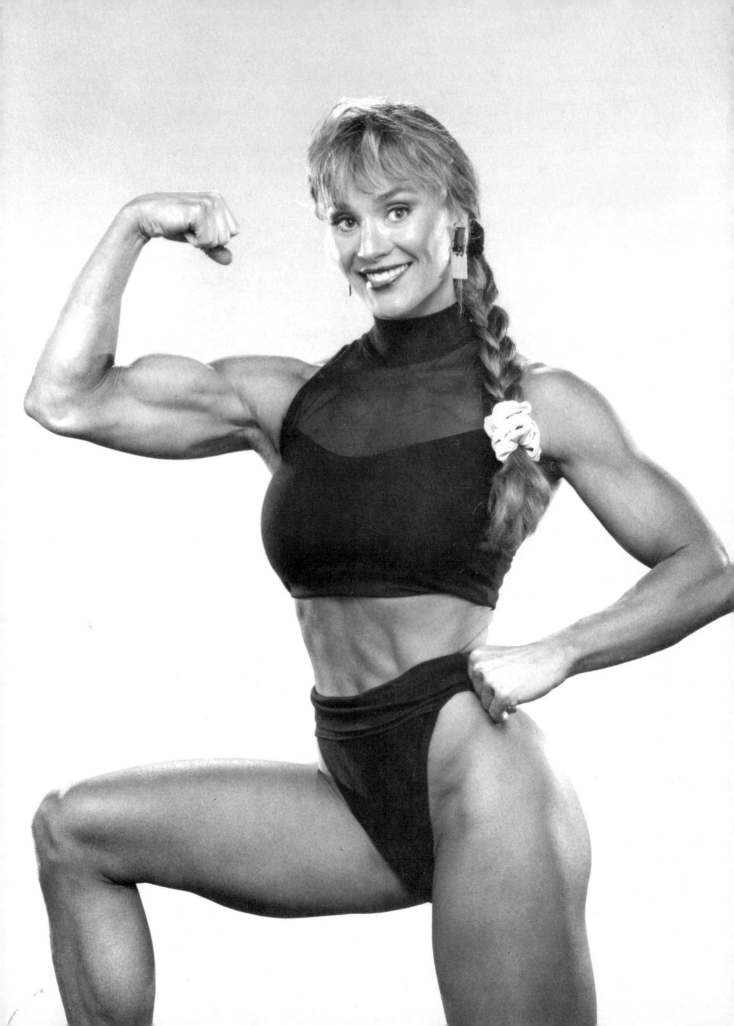

Three

Dieters Beware: It's a Jungle Out There!

Are you trying to lose weight? Watch out! There's a quack around every corner peddling magical cures and potions to banish fat. If only it were that easy!

During the decade I was a professional bodybuilder, I was forced to maintain my weight and fat level at unrealistically low levels. I was continually assaulted by—and at times even tempted to try—quickie weight-loss gimmicks. What woman could turn down a pill that blocks the absorption of starch so you could eat to your heart's content—without ever gaining an ounce? And who wouldn't trade endless situps for a magical cream that miraculously melts away fat?

I soon discovered that if it sounded too good to be true, it usually was—except for the advertisers making all the money.

FAT GONE WRONG?

To save you the time, trouble, and expense of using yourself as a guinea pig, let's dismiss some of the most common myths about weight loss, beginning with a term that's been around for years: cellulite.

You know what we're talking about: that quivers-when-you-walk stuff that clings to your hips, thighs, and buttocks and gives you dimples where you least want them. (And which we attempt to camouflage with long T-shirts, the fashion statement of the overweight or amply endowed.)

But before you invest your next paycheck on products or treatments that promise to banish this alleged hard-to-budge pudge, whether it's an herbal wrap that "sets fat free" or hip boots that squeeze your fat into hiding, there's something you should know about cellulite. It's just another name for plain old fat.

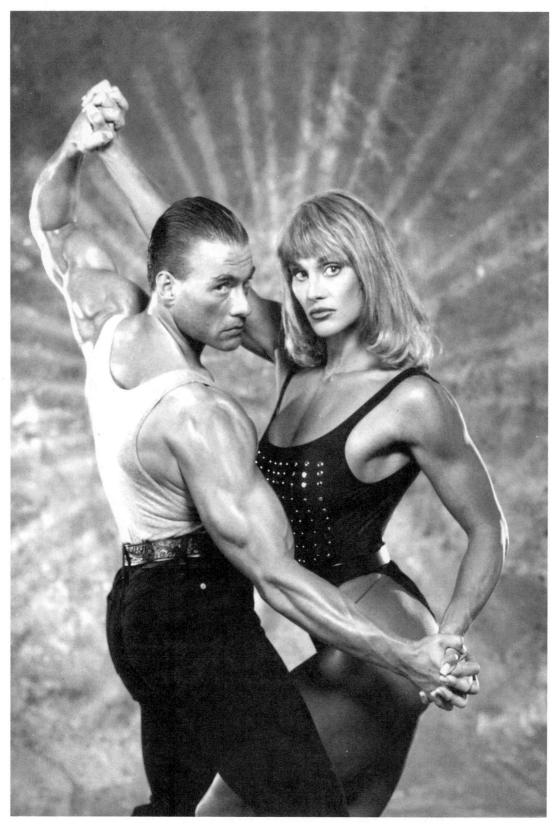

As a professional bodybuilder, staying in shape was my full-time profession. It landed me a role in my very first movie, *Double Impact*.

In fact the American Medical Association states flatly that there is no medical condition known or described as cellulite. The FDA describes the condition known as cellulite as "fat on fat"—double-decker fat, but fat nonetheless.

Unfortunately, the myth of cellulite continues to be perpetrated by a slew of anti-cellulite fad diets, spot-reducing exercises, wraps, packs, and massages which can only be dismissed as thigh-in-the-sky wishful thinking. Maybe, as *Shape* magazine once suggested, they should spell it Sell-U-Lite instead?

As women age, certain outer skin layers get thinner and elastic, which is why quivering thighs start showing up in the 40-something crowd. Meanwhile, all guys get is a beer belly—and distinguished gray hair.

PLAIN OLD FAT

Scientists believe the rippling effect is caused by a network of connective tissue fibers that attach muscle to skin and compartmentalize the fat, like stitching on a quilt. The more stuffing there is, the more puckered the texture, so even the thinnest layer of padding may not lie flat.

It's true that some women—and most—men—sail through life cellulite-free, even when they gain weight. Chalk it up to chromosomal differences.

Unaware of the role of genetics, women have tried everything from creams to liposuction to rid themselves of cellulite. For an imaginary condition, cellulite certainly is persistent!

HIT PARADE OF QUACK CURES

From worthless to bogus creams, William Jarvis, Ph.D., president of the National Council Against Health Fraud and a professor of health education at Loma Linda University, has seen it all. Disguised as a willing dupe, he travels the "health quack circuit" incognito, using himself as a guinea pig.

Here are a few of the more common cellulite cures Jarvis has documented:

Cellulite Wraps

During this popular spa treatment, you're wrapped King Tut-fashion and set aside for an hour to steam away your fat. Falling for this bum "wrap" may be dangerous because tightly wrapping the body can lead to dehydration or to serious complications for those with diabetes or varicose veins.

Cellulite Massage

Hands off this hands-on remedy. Proponents claim it pounds away at cellulite, breaking it down so that it's easily eliminated by the body. But while massage can relax and stimulate muscles and help push metabolic wastes on their way, it can't burn off fat. The only person who's getting a workout during massage is the therapist. Fat cells, like tissues, can't be moved unless you get them "Hoovered" out via liposuction. They can only shrink or grow in place.

Cellulite Scrubbers

Here's an interesting take on the dental plaque advertisements. Don't bank on it. No matter how hard you scrub with brushes, horsehair mats, and other garbage sold for this purpose, the only thing you'll remove is the top layer (or maybe more) of your skin while the fat will continue to sit pretty seven floors below.

Dream-On Creams

The latest cure for cellulite comes in a tube, according to every cosmetics company putting out a cream or gel. But because of complaints from the medical community and FDA, companies have been forced to reword their claims to state that the creams do not actually reduce or eliminate cellulite but merely improve the way it looks. Unfortunately, the message often gets lost in the selling. While these creams contain emollients and preservatives that might plump up the skin with moisturizers, the smoothing effect is only temporary.

All-Natural Vitamins, Supplements, Etc.

The supplements contain diuretics that drain your body of needed water for a temporarily slimmer look. As soon as you drink a glass of water, back comes the "cellulite."

Passive Fat-Zappers

If only it were true. We could close the gyms of the world, melt down the stair climbers and barbells and recycle them into something more useful, then lie down and vibrate our fat away. Proponents claim vibrating machines are as effective as 1,000 situps. Yeah, sure. Then why are all these cellulite-infested women still on the planet?

Hormone and Enzyme Injections

Don't let anyone stick you with this stuff, which could be anything from sugar water to cow gland extract. Whatever they put in the syringe doesn't work.

Summing up the cellulite scam, Jarvis says, "You'll save yourself thousands of dollars and possibly physical injury by seeing cellulite for what it is—an illusion created by hucksters who couldn't care less about taking away your fat. The only thing they want to take away is your money."

LIPOSUCTION

Talk about a modern-day miracle-maker. You go to sleep, a surgeon inserts a few tubes, switches on his Hoover, and you wake up cellulite-free forever—from pudgy to svelte in an hour flat.

If only it were so. Unfortunately, Virginia, the surgery vacuums only deeper fat, not the surface layer responsible for the dappling, and this can actually make cellulite look worse. Some surgeons are experimenting with a new technique which involves cutting fibrous connective cords, removing excess fat from the superficial layer, and then reinjecting a little fat liposuctioned from another part of the body to even things out, but don't hold your breath. Not only is the procedure expensive—one New York surgeon charges $2,500 to $4,000 for the job—but no one can promise the connective cords won't grow back or that the injected fat won't dance around or otherwise misbehave.

While plastic surgeons once insisted that fat cells never grow back once they're removed, Thomas Wadden, Ph.D., director of the Center for Health and Behavior at Syracuse University, says new studies show otherwise. Over a period of time, fat cells may regenerate or cause ad-jacent fat cells to expand in number to match an individualized set point for body fat. In other words, if you remove what your body perceives to be its normal number of fat cells. it will re-place them with new ones until its former quota is reached.

Which isn't to say that liposuction doesn't have merit for a selected group of women. Let's say you're in great shape with one blaring exception. You have saddlebags that could beat the Pony Express. Not only do they camouflage an otherwise great pair of legs but they give you an unfashionably lopsided look and a bad body image. Meanwhile, you've done everything under the sun to get rid of them, including running long-distance marathons. The last time you won a 10-K, they were right there with you—loyal to the end. You may be a perfect candidate for liposuction. On the other hand . . .

Liposuction is neither a universal panacea for being overweight, nor a substitute for diet and exercise. It will never make a fat woman thin. Rather, it's a refining process during which one to two pounds of excess padding are removed from a specific area of the body to give an otherwise fit physique better balance and contour. Put simply, liposuction makes all your parts match and can enhance self-confidence, leading to a healthier body image and thus even elim-inate eating disorders—provided it's done on the right person.

Garth Fisher, M.D., and John William, M.D., both certified plastic surgeons with Aesthetica in Beverly Hills, define a "good" candidate for liposuction as a healthy woman of normal weight who has fat pads on her hips, thighs, buttocks, or abdomen that resist all realistic diet and ex-ercise programs. (By realistic, we mean healthful diets and an exercise program you can fit into your daily life; exercising nine hours a day would undoubtedly banish every bulge from your body, but who has the time or energy for that?) That is, while a woman with excess flab may need six months to diet and exercise off excess fat, a woman with inherited pockets may literally be stuck with them—no matter what she does.

Those who don't qualify are women who are overweight or obese by their own doing. They refuse to adhere to a diet or exercise program and view surgery as a quick fix, sometimes to their entire lives.

And buyer beware, cautions most reputable plastic surgeons. The hefty cost of liposuction has attracted a large number of disreputable practitioners who perform the operation without proper training, experience, or credentials, and the medical journals are full of horror stories. Before considering liposuction, seek out the advice of a well-trained, qualified plastic surgeon who is board-certified in plastic surgery—not pediatrics, pharmacology, or career counseling. Nor-mally, most patients experience bruising and swelling following surgery, with recovery time last-ing a few weeks or so, depending on how much fat was removed. But mix a poor candidate with an unqualified surgeon and horrendous complications may occur, from bleeding, infection, numbness, unsightly rippling, and discoloration to death.

LIPOSUCTION TO REDUCE APPLE-TYPE RISKS?

If you think you may qualify for liposuction, choose a surgeon who is qualified by the American Board of Plastic Surgeons and who has additional training in the procedure. But promise me just one thing. Don't even think about it until you've given my diet and exercise program an honest chance—at least six months. It may take a little longer than liposuction, but it lasts forever—and you won't turn black and blue in the process!

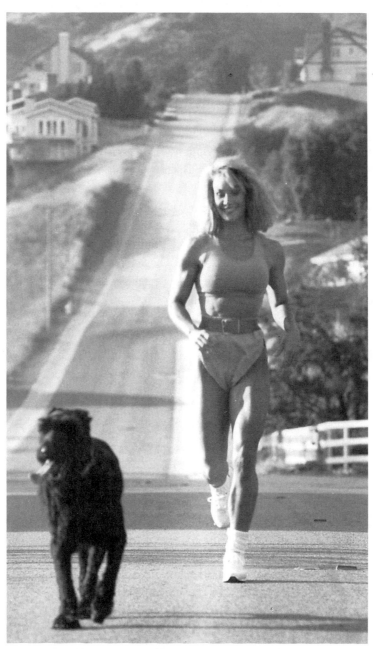

Don't let quick-fix cons steer you away from a healthful exercise program. My fitness buddy, Bolaro, makes sure I don't skip out on fitness. He's always on time and ready to go.

FAD DIETS MAKE YOU FAT

We've already discussed the metabolic nightmare that chronic dieting sets in motion: The less you eat, the lower you drive down your metabolism until finally, you could almost live on air. Some people gain weight eating just 500 calories a day because they've trained their bodies to be ultra-conservative.

When your body senses starvation, it clamps down and burns every available calorie very carefully—and slooooowly.

BAD NEWS DIETS

Any diet is bad news, but some commercial ones have made a fine science out of manipulating the public into adopting ridiculous and possibly dangerous eating habits.

You've heard them all: from diets that ban *all* foods to those that revolve around an al- leged wonder food: bananas, rice, seaweed, yogurt, grapefruit . . .

Regardless of which ploy they use to sell you, these diets all have one thing in common: They don't work! You may loose weight temporarily, but let's face it. Woman cannot live on grapefruit alone. The minute you try to eat normally, wham! Those pounds creep back faster than you can say "food-combining"—which is another totally bogus concept.

Take a close look at what these diets allow you to eat and it's actually a blessing that few can stomach them for longer than a few weeks, as most are dangerously unbalanced nutrition- ally.

So we'd like to offer a description of the general categories of bad news diets. We're sure you'll be able to locate your favorite flop among them.

THE WORLD'S WORST DIETS

High-protein Diets

These high-protein, low-carbohydrate diets ban bread, cereal, and limit fruits and vegetables on the grounds they are fattening, and push dairy products that are high in saturated animal fats and cholesterol. Many of these diets also include marginal levels of important nutrients, such as vitamins A and C, thiamine, riboflavin, and niacin. And their high-fat content may be a heart attack waiting to happen, not to mention what they could do to your blood cholesterol. Because of the abnormally-high level of protein, these diets force your kidneys to get rid of large amounts of nitrogen waste and may contribute to calcium and bone loss.

Quick Weight-Loss Or Water Diets

Also low in carbohydrates and high in protein and fat, these diets rob your body of calcium, vitamins A, C, and thiamine. And with little fruit, vegetables, or grains or roughage, they're also likely to leave you constipated.

Low-Carbohydrate Diets

These diets limit fats and include some fruits and vegetables, but they are far too low in carbohydrates and too high in protein to be healthful. Besides, these diets are totally retro, a throwback to the dietary Dark Ages when the kindly if unenlightened family doc—who hadn't cracked a medical journal in years—poked a tubby finger at your tummy bulge, called it a "bread basket," and advised you to lay off the starch. For 15 years, my coauthor ate less bread than a prisoner in maximum security until someone finally assured her that it wasn't fattening.

As for me, I live on carbs and I dare you to find a bread basket on me anywhere!

Rice-Only Type Diets

Diets that exclude food groups are bad news. Without fruits and vegetables, you could develop vitamin deficiencies. Besides, in this world of infinite choices, we have trouble staying married to the same person for life, much less eating the same food at every meal.

Low-Protein Diets

These diets rule out nearly all protein, which may lead to calcium and iron deficiencies, which in turn will cause you to lose muscle—your most valuable fat-burner.

Sure, you may wind up looking slimmer, but you'll actually be "fatter," that is, you'll have a higher percentage of fat to muscle than before, and your metabolism will take a beating that could take years to repair.

Liquid Diets

These Spartan regimens call for 200 to 400 calories daily in the form of liquid-protein preparations. The theory here is that by ignoring real food, you won't be tempted to eat it.

That's fine if you live on the moon. Otherwise, you'd better beat a path that avoids all kitchens, and restaurants, and bakeries, and fast food joints . . .

Food Combining

This diet calls for eating designated groups of foods in specific combinations on the preposterous medical assumption that it is somehow possible to slow down the normal digestive process by eating foods in combination.

Because it inhibits the complete absorption of food and has so little protein, it eventually leads to exhaustion and even anemia. Follow this diet for long and you won't be fit for much of anything—except sleeping—especially if you follow it religiously which advocates claim is essential for the diet to "work."

Vegetarianism/Macrobiotics/Vegan Diets

All three diets are inherently healthful if you follow them to the letter and create complete proteins by combining legumes, beans, and rice. Unfortunately, many women simply cut the beef and never master the substitutes. In the process, they rob their bodies of essential vitamins, minerals, and proteins needed to build, maintain, and repair bodily tissues, muscles, bones, skin, and hair. I know this trap firsthand, having winged it for years as a vegetarian before buckling down and learning how to combine beans, legumes, and rice to make complete proteins. For more on eating a balanced vegetarian diet, see Chapters 4 and 5.

WASTED NUTRIENTS

Fad diets, in addition to ruining your metabolism, encouraging obesity and, robbing you of vital nutrients, can also throw your absorption process out of kilter. According to Nancy R. Stevenson, Ph.D., of the University of Medicine and Dentistry of New Jersey–Robert Wood Johnson Medical School, people on low-fat diets may have reduced capacity to absorb fat-soluble vitamins such as vitamins A, D, E, and beta-carotene. Poor retention of one vitamin often results in a domino effect, so you lose others, too. For instance, if you can't absorb vitamin D, you may not be able to absorb calcium properly, which could lead to bone problems later in life. General and cosmetic dentist Steven Donia, D.D.S., of Northridge, California, sees a loss of bone density, not only in older women with osteoporosis, but also in 14–30 year olds with eating disorders, and this loss is caused by a lack of essential vitamins and minerals in their diet.

While supplements may sound like the logical solution, if improperly taken, they can do more harm than good: High doses of zinc, vitamin C, or fructose can interfere with copper absorption, while too much vitamin E can block proper absorption of beta-carotene.

TEN TIPOFFS TO A BAD DIET

Avoid a weight-loss program like the plague if it falls into any of these categories.

1. Eliminates a basic food group (all dairy, or all fruits, or all meat, poultry, fish, legumes or tofu, or all breads and grains).
2. Calls for a drastic reduction in complex carbohydrates (cereal, grains, breads), fruits and vegetables.
3. Provides less than 1,000 calories a day.
4. Revolves around a liquid diet.
5. Bans all snacks.
6. Revolves around one or two foods, no matter how healthful those foods may be (e.g., rice).
7. Forces you to buy exotic or hard-to-get foods.
8. Revolves around prepackaged powders or expensive supplements.
9. Dismisses the importance of exercise or has no exercise component.
10. Promotes expensive herbal or "natural" remedies on grounds that they "burn" fat.

OTHER USELESS DIET GIMMICKS

Water Pills and Diuretics

Rather than helping you lose weight, all these pills do is dehydrate you—often dangerously so. Although you may lose up to 10 pounds by taking them, as soon you drink water the pounds come back. Water pills can also result in improper muscle functioning and may disrupt your nor-

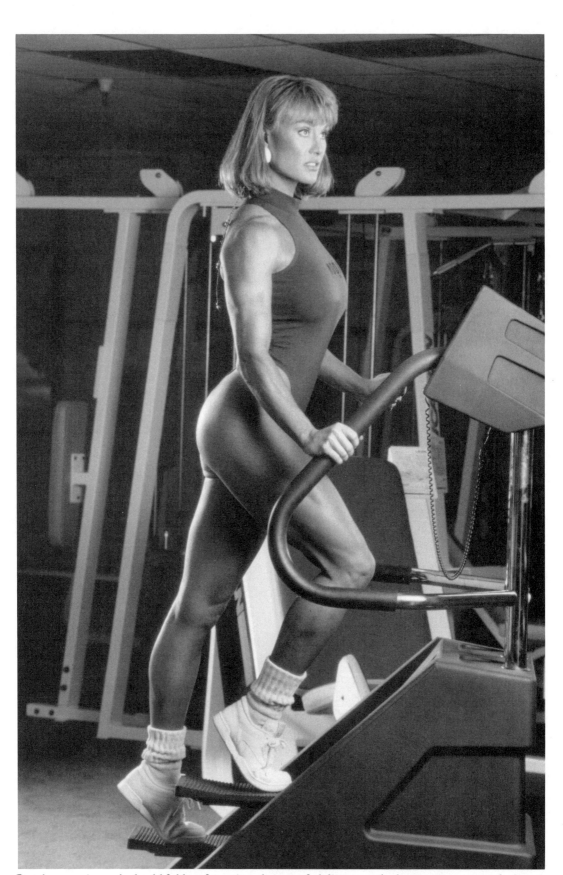

Regular exercise and a healthful low-fat eating plan—not fad diets—are the key to success, so take it one step at a time.

mal balance of salts, which can make you lightheaded or dizzy. While sometimes prescribed for specific health problems such as high blood pressure or congestive heart failure, they aren't for casual use to eliminate bloating or promote weight loss. They are medicine and should never be taken without a doctor's orders.

Laxatives

You can flush this one down the toilet, too. As with water pills, laxatives are bad news for dieters. Again, what you lose is water, not fat, as most laxatives simply increase the water in your stools so you eliminate food faster. While the passage may be so fast that sometimes food is not absorbed, you rarely "lose" enough calories to justify the risks.

Laxative abuse also interferes with the absorption of essential vitamins and minerals like potassium. And laxatives can become addictive and eventually cripple your bowel muscle function, leading to chronic constipation.

Fiber Pills

Generally swallowed before meals to create a feeling of fullness to encourage you to eat less, fiber pills are not so much dangerous as unnecessary. Why not just drink a few glasses of water for the same feeling of fullness? Skip the pills and do as I do and rise and shine to a bowl of bran cereal with fresh fruit sliced on top. It's a tasty way to start your day—and you'll never have to worry again about being regular.

Appetite Suppressants Or "Diet Pills"

These include phenylpropoanolamine and amphetamines. Both are prescription drugs that may reduce your appetite. But both are highly addictive and not worth the health risks—regardless of how much weight you need to lose. Because they stimulate the nervous system, they are likely to make you feel jittery, nervous, irritable and may interfere with your normal sleep cycle. And once you stop taking them, you're likely to quickly regain the weight.

As for the growing line of over-the-counter diet pills, there's no medical evidence that they help people lose weight.

Thyroid Pills

If your thyroid is normal, thyroid pills can't facilitate weight loss; Your thyroid will simply cut back on its production of hormones. And people who do lose weight lose lean muscle mass, not fat.

HCG (Human Chorionic Gonadrotrophin)

HCG, a hormone produced by the placenta which is made from the urine of pregnant women, is prescribed by disreputable weight-loss clinics in conjunction with a very low-calorie diet. Studies show that it's the diet, not HCG, that accounts for weight loss. Frankly, just thinking about consuming this stuff is enough to make me lose my appetite—or my cookies. (Maybe that's why it works.) What will these hucksters think up next? Bottling spider webs and selling them as a diet aid?

Intestinal Bypass

As with liposuction, this is a last resort for the obese and involves surgically bypassing a part of the small intestine to reduce food absorption. Although the surgery can lead to serious complications, including severe diarrhea and liver problems, it has proven successful in cases involving very overweight people.

Herbal Remedies

The problem with herbs is that no long-term studies have been conducted to show what they do, and there are no standards of purity. Just because it's natural (so is uranium) doesn't mean it's safe—or that it will help you lose weight.

SHOULD YOU JOIN A GROUP?

Commercial weight-loss organizations may be a helpful crutch for those who have the wish but lack the willpower and/or knowledge to lose weight safely.

They may also be ideal for those who lose weight best in a structured, monitored setting with weekly group support, weigh-ins, and a day-by-day, detailed, down-to-the-last-calorie meal plan.

Unfortunately, not all weight-loss clinics are legitimate. Even the best, medically approved commercial chains may offer inconsistent quality of service. The worst of the worst serve as mere fronts for expensive, low-calorie meals that cost four times more than what you would pay for the same food in supermarkets. Do your homework before signing on the dotted line. You could lose more money and time than weight.

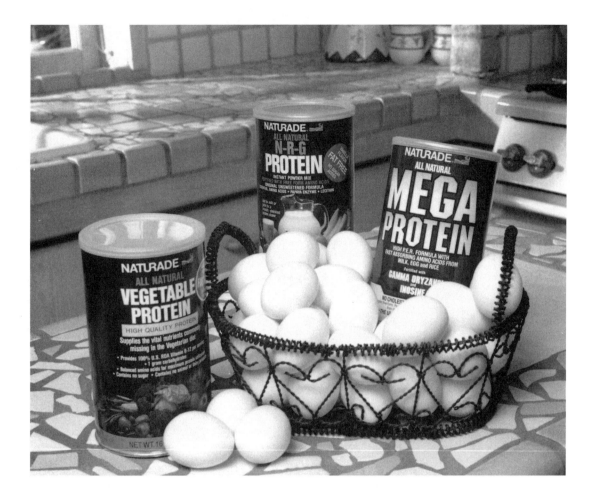

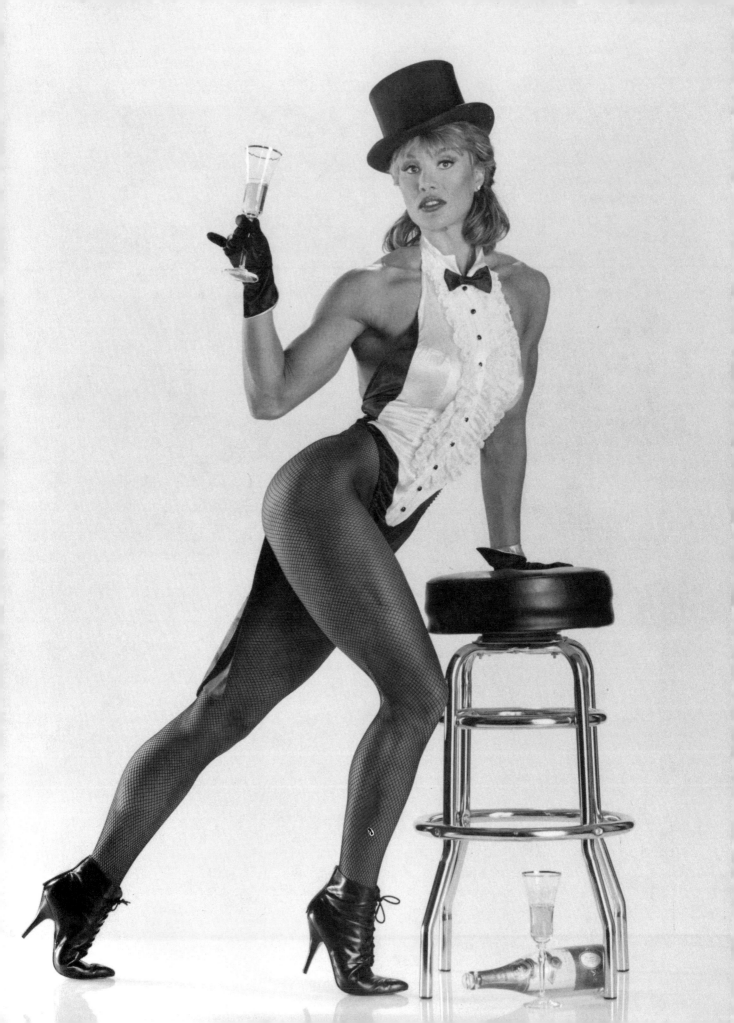

Four

Eat More, Lose More

Remember when starch was considered the dietary villain, and we gobbled down bacon and eggs believing this was a healthful breakfast?

A lot has changed since then, beginning with the Basic Four Food Groups we grew up with. You remember—that food chart with the smiling cheeses and dancing milk cartons that hung on our grade-school walls?

The fact is, the Basic Four isn't so basic anymore. We know much more about nutrition than we did in the 1950s. A few years ago, the U.S. Department of Agriculture unveiled the Food Guide Pyramid, a brand-new national food plan based on the latest nutrition research that reshuffles our dietary priorities and relegates the Basic Four to the Dark Ages. The Basic Four gave equal importance to meat, dairy products, grain products, and fruits, and vegetables, calling for four servings of each.

The Pyramid puts grains on a pedestal, suggesting that we eat 6 to 11 servings daily, while decreasing the amount of dairy and red meat products to 2 to 3 servings.

MATTER OF FAT

Why? It's all a matter of fat. Meat and dairy products pack far more fat than grains, fruits, and vegetables. Not that we don't need some dairy and meat—and even some fat—every day. But current research shows we need a lot less than we once believed.

In fact, according to nutrition experts, the pyramid represents the first truly healthy eating plan this country has ever had—not counting native Americans who had the nutrition smarts all along with their primarily grain diet.

Frankly, I'm delighted that the masses are following the sort of eating habits that have powered professional athletes for years. Bring on the pasta, bread, grains, vegetables, and fruits! And easy on the meat, dairy products, and most of all, fat.

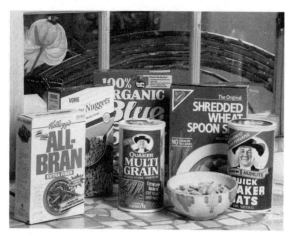

So long, bacon and eggs. Today's healthful breakfast is more likely to center around whole-grain cereals and breads.

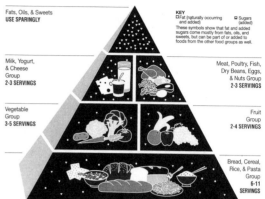

Food Pyramid

JUST ENOUGH INFO TO BE DANGEROUS

So why the sudden turnaround from bacon and eggs to oatmeal and beans? The impetus for a new national food plan began in the late 1970s. Increasing evidence linked excess fat to heart disease, breast cancer, and other diseases and made it clear that the Basic Four, which contains great big gobs of greasy, grimy fat from dairy products and meat, needed a major overhaul.

Because the Basic Four was so vague as to what exact foods you *should* choose within each of the four food groups, you could pick hot dogs instead of lean beef, ice cream instead of non-fat yogurt, French fries instead of broccoli—and score an A+ for good nutrition. Unfortunately, that's exactly what a lot of Americans did. How do you think McDonald's sold a billion burgers? Not only did the Basic Four lead us astray, but it gave us just enough information to be dangerous.

In 1989, the USDA assembled a committee of independent nutritionists to develop new national dietary guidelines that would reflect the latest findings on nutrition and the dangers of fat. Unlike the Basic Four, which gave all foods equal billing, the pyramid showed at a glance that foods that come from plants—not animals—should be the basis of our diet.

My diet is as close to this as I can get within my sanity range; in fact, to compensate for my daily Snickers bar, I'm as strict as a monk the rest of the day and eat hardly any fat at all.

NOT PERFECT YET

While a good start, the pyramid is by no means picture perfect. It doesn't provide enough information about what foods to eat and avoid within a specific food group. It also lumps healthy and fatty foods together in one group, which can be confusing.

Rather than reprinting the government pyramid, we've taken the pyramid and expanded it to show you the best and worst foods to eat by food group. That way, you won't be eating French fries when you should be eating baked potatoes—hold the butter!

SEVEN GOLDEN RULES

The Pyramid Food Guide is really just a visual representation of the USDA's seven new dietary guidelines:

1. Eat a variety of foods.
2. Maintain a healthy weight.
3. Choose a diet low in fat, saturated fat, and cholesterol.
4. Choose a diet with plenty of vegetables, fruits, and grain products.
5. Use sugars only in moderation.
6. Use salt and sodium only in moderation, especially if you have high blood pressure.
7. If you drink alcoholic beverages, do so in moderation.

Pretty simple, huh?

PUTTING THE PYRAMID TOGETHER

If you're a meat and dairy queen, it's time to revamp your diet and think breads, grains, and starches.

To repeat: STARCHES DO NOT MAKE YOU FAT. FAT MAKES YOU FAT. So load up on starches and consider meat and dairy products as pinch hitters to be eaten sparingly.

Remember that you need a little from each food group so don't eliminate one.

AMAZING GRAINS

Whole-grain breads and grains are a low-fat source of time-released energy, and they provide fiber, which helps control weight, promotes regularity, and satisfies hunger. They also supply large amounts of the three key B vitamins, and iron. Because they are stored as glycogen in muscles, complex carbohydrates found in all grain products are also critical for endurance sports.

How much we need: Six to 11 servings daily. One serving equals 1 slice of bread, 1 ounce of ready-to-eat cereal or ½ cup cooked cereal, rice, or pasta. Don't panic—as you can see, it only sounds like a lot. Fill your cereal bowl or eat a plate of pasta and you've already consumed two to four servings.

Fill 'er Up: Great choices include breads, bagels, pita, muffins, biscuits, and buns with less than 2 grams of fat per serving; cold cereals with less than 2 grams of fat and less than 6 grams of sugar per serving (e.g., Cheerios, corn flakes, shredded wheat, Grape Nuts.); crackers with less than one gram of fat per half ounce: Melba toast, matzoh, flatbread, saltines.

Also, hot cereals: (e.g. oatmeal, Cream of Wheat); non- or low-fat crackers, cakes, pastries, cookies, and other desserts; unbuttered, air-popped popcorn, pretzels, rice cakes, breadsticks, corn tortillas.

Eat less: Bread stuffing, crackers with more than 3 grams of fat per half ounce, high-fat pastries, cakes, croissants, muffins, biscuits, and breads with more than 4 grams of fat per serving, oil-popped or buttered popcorn. Remember: just about anything on the shelves with fat can be found or prepared without fat.

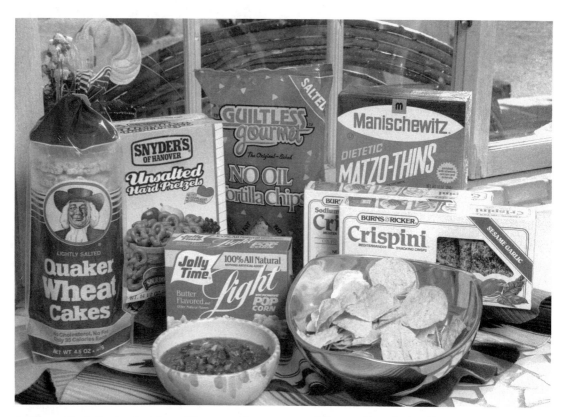

Just keep the fattening toppings—like peanut butter—to a minimum. Cereals, breads, and crackers are an important source of carbohydrates. Try the new low- and non-fat products and you'll cut down on extra fat as well.

EAT YOUR VEGETABLES

I can't live without them! Do as I do and take a bag of frozen vegetables, toss the entire bag in the microwave, yank them out, season with herbs or a dab of olive oil and voila! A meal in a minute. (No wonder my boyfriend's mother is concerned . . .)

Vegetables are naturally low-fat, high-fiber foods that are high in vitamins A and C as well as the minerals folate, iron, and magnesium.

How much we need: The pyramid recommends that we eat 3 to 5 servings daily. One serving equals 1 cup of raw leafy vegetables, ½ cup cooked or raw vegetables, or ¾ cup vegetable juice.

Fill 'er Up: Best choices include all fresh vegetables, dark-green leafy vegetables such as spinach, romaine, and broccoli (high in vitamins and minerals), starchy vegetables, including carrots, squash, corn and potatoes (high in fiber).

Eat less: Fresh or frozen vegetables in sauces and salads with heavy or mayonnaise-based sauces, such as potato salad and cole slaw.

FRUITS TO THE RESCUE

Fruits and fruit juices are low in fat and sodium and provide ample amounts of vitamins A and C, potassium, and fiber. This is my favorite category; I could eat fruit all day!

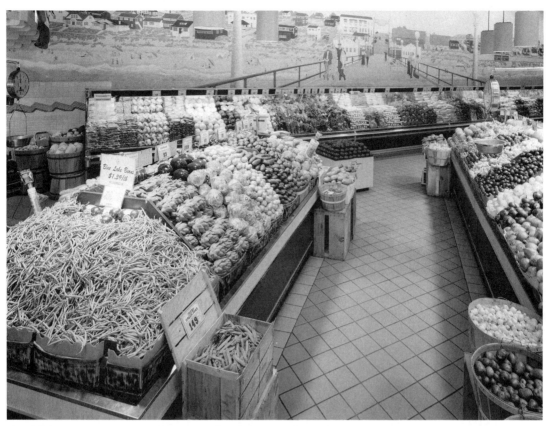

One of the most important aisles in your local supermarket is the produce department, so roll your cart by and stock up.

How much we need: The pyramid recommends 2 to 4 servings daily. One serving equals 1 medium apple, banana, or orange; ½ cup of chopped, cooked, or canned fruit, or ¾ cup of fruit juice.

Fill 'er Up: Great choices are all fresh fruit except avocados and olives; citrus fruits, berries, and melons (especially high in vitamin C); unsweetened fruit juices.

Eat less: Avocados, canned or frozen fruit in heavy syrup; dried fruit, olives, sweetened applesauce.

DON'T BE A MEATHEAD

Most of us already eat too much protein; the excess turns into fat, so why overdose on it? We do need some, as meat, poultry, and fish supply B vitamins, iron, and zinc. Dried beans, eggs, and nuts provide protein and many, but not all, of the vitamins and minerals found in meat, and, unfortunately, not nearly as much as once thought.

How much we need: The food pyramid recommends 2 to 3 servings, with one serving equaling 2 to 3 ounces of cooked lean meat, poultry or fish, ½ cup cooked dry beans, 1 egg or 2 tablespoons of peanut butter for each ounce of lean meat (less than 3 grams of fat per ounce).

Fill 'er Up: In the bean department, stock up on dried beans, peas, and lentils, navy, pinto, kidney beans, and chickpeas, which can be used in place of meat. Egg whites also are high in protein.

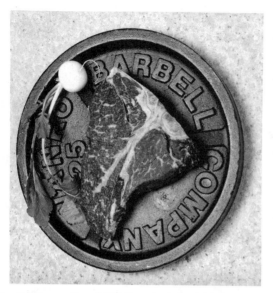

Don't be a meathead. While some is healthful, too much will weigh you down and turn to fat—not muscle.

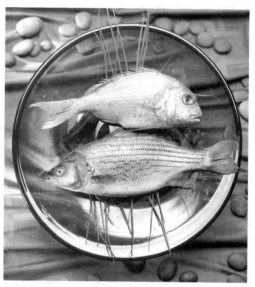

Fish is a tasty and low-fat form of protein. Eat it several times a week if you can, instead of meat.

Fresh fish is a low-fat winner. Broil, roast, or boil rather than fry or grill it.

In the red meat category, choose round, loin, sirloin, chuck arm cuts of beef. For pork, go with tenderloin, center loin, or ham. For lamb, the foreshank is best. All types of veal are fine except ground, which tends to be fatty.

In the poultry department, choose breast, leg, and wing and always cooked without the skin, which traps a high percentage of the fat.

For lean lunching, try the new line of low-fat deli meats and water-canned tuna.

Eat less: Meats with more than 3 grams of fat per ounce, including bacon, bologna, brisket, chuck blade roast, corned beef, frankfurters, ground beef, liver, pastrami, porterhouse steak, rib-eye, ribs, short ribs. Also, all duck and goose, regular deli meats, nuts, seeds and nut butters and whole eggs or egg yolks. (My mother used to spread goose grease on top of rye bread, an unappetizing or questionable German "delicacy" that makes my fat cells dance.)

DRINK YOUR MILK?

Remember when your mother made you drink a full glass of whole milk with every meal? Come on, Mom, get hip! While we certainly need some dairy products for calcium and to supply other vitamins and minerals needed for strong bones and teeth, a little goes a long way. The pyramid recommends 2 to 3 servings a day; one serving equals 1 cup milk or yogurt, 1½ ounces natural cheese, or 2 ounces processed cheese.

Fill 'er Up: Great choices are low- or non-fat cheese, cottage cheese, milk and yogurt; cheeses with less than 2 grams of fat per half cup; frozen dairy desserts and ice milk and frozen yogurt with less than 2 grams of fat per half-cup serving.

Eat/drink less: Whole milk, cheese containing more than 5 grams of fat per ounce, including creamed and cottage cheeses, hot cocoa or chocolate milk made from 2 percent milk, ice cream and frozen dairy desserts with more than 5 grams of fat per half-cup serving, puddings made with whole milk and yogurt made from whole milk.

HOLD THE LINE ON FAT

We all need a little. But there is soooo much hidden fat in nearly everything we eat that we don't have to even think about adding any. As for me, a Snickers bar more than fulfills my daily fat quota.

Fats provide warmth for our bodies, are essential for healthy skin and energy, carry fat-soluble vitamins, and line internal organs, while simple sugars (table sugar, brown sugar, honey) and sweets offer few nutrients but provide quick energy. Again, a little goes a long way, as fats and oils contain more than twice the calories found in carbohydrates and sugar supplies little if any vitamins or minerals.

How much we need: Limit fat to 20 to 30 percent of total daily calories and sugar to 24 to 72 grams daily, depending on your exercise and activity level.

Fill 'er up: Great choices include non- or low-fat margarine or spreads, non- or low-fat salad dressing, and monosaturated fats found mostly in canola, peanut and olive oil. Monounsaturated fats raise HDL (good cholesterol) and lower LDL (bad cholesterol). Also, un-saturated vegetable oils and margarine that list a liquid vegetable oil as the first ingredient on the label.

Eat less: Products containing large amounts of saturated or partially hydrogenated fats such as butter, cakes, cookies, ice cream, non-dairy creamers, pastries, and pie crusts.

FIND YOUR SERVING RANGE

The Pyramid provides a range of caloric intake and servings based on activity level. The USDA recommends that if you're a couch potato or exercise less than three times weekly (tsk! get moving!), follow the lowest range. If you exercise at least three times weekly for 30 minutes, use the moderate range. If you exercise regularly (backpacking, cross-country skiing, mountain biking, long-distance cycling, in-line skating, running, triathlons, etc.), or are training for a marathon or trying to gain weight, follow the high range. Feel free to alternate between ranges depending on your activity level.

FOCUS ON STARCH

Now that you understand what the new food pyramid is all about, let's take a closer look at the new building block of our diet—complex carbohydrates, or what we once called "starch."

Remember when people—even doctors—thought starches were fattening? I remember my mother telling me to be careful of eating too much or I'd get fat.

Today, my diet remains about 70 percent starch and 30 percent or less protein, exactly what I ate to build large muscles and strength as a professional bodybuilder. I must admit I de-voured mounds of spinach in hopes of resembling a female Popeye.

For the average woman who wants pretty, feminine muscles, a high-protein diet is not nec-essary and, in fact, is likely to make you fatter, not more muscular. Many protein foods such

	SEDENTARY	ACTIVE	VERY ACTIVE
Calories	1,600	2,200	2,800
Bread Servings	6	9	5
Vegetable	3	4	5
Fruit	2	3	4
Milk	2 to 3*	2 to 3*	2 to 3*
Meat	2	2	3
	(total 5 oz)	(total 6 oz)	(total 7 oz)
Total fat			
(grams)	53	73	93
Total added sugar	6	12	18
(grams; 4 grams = 1 teaspoon)			

*Pregnant women and nursing mothers should use the higher figure.

as meat and dairy products are high in fat. Pig out on protein and the excess won't be stored as muscle but as plain old fat. Most of us get enough protein without trying to eat more—too much, in fact—while few people eat too much carbohydrate.

Meanwhile, if you want to lose pounds, a high-carbohydrate diet helps you maintain your weight and health by providing more power with less fat than any other food. Starches don't make you fat—fat does. One teaspoon of carbohydrate has only 16 calories compared to 36 calories per teaspoon of fat. And carbs take more energy to convert to fat. Our bodies need only three percent of the ingested calories to convert dietary fat into body fat, whereas to convert excess carbohydrates into fat requires 23 percent of the ingested calories.

Studies show that people fed high-fat diets gained weight more easily than those who eat high-carbohydrate diets. Those who ate a standard diet but consumed extra calories in fat gained the same amount of weight in three months as was gained in seven months by people who consumed the same amount of extra calories in carbohydrates. In other words, if you eat something with a high fat content, it is much easier to store that fat on your hips, thighs, and butt because it is already fat in a storeable state. Carbohydrates, on the other hand, need to be converted into fat to be stored—and that conversion requires calories.

And because carbohydrates are filling and take more energy to digest, they also tend to stick with you. For instance, a bowl of rice will take longer to digest and keep you feeling fuller longer than, say, a bowl of ice cream. Since carbohydrate calories are less fattening than fat calories, you can eat far more without gaining weight. Carbs are also usually high in fiber, which creates a feeling of fullness so you eat less.

Complex carbohydrates are also our best sources of time-released, long-term energy. A high-carb diet gives you lots of energy. Remember when carbo-loading was a big deal, with runners and cyclists gobbling down huge plates of spaghetti or starches before a race to give them extra get-up-and-go? Experts today recommend eating lots of starches all the time—even if you never intend to run a race.

Research shows diets high in soluble fiber found in breads and grains may help lower blood cholesterol, thus helping prevent heart disease.

Finally, carbs help control blood-sugar levels. In many cases, diabetics have been able to reduce or eliminate their requirements for drugs or insulin, becoming non-insulin dependent diabetics.

As for me, lead me to the bagels, the pasta, the spaghetti. My friends joke that I'm one of the few people they know who could live quite happily on a prisoner's diet of bread and water. Throw in some jelly beans and Snickers and lock me away!

You probably already have plenty of carbs in your kitchen cupboards—bread, bagels, noodles, pasta, breakfast cereals, potatoes, rice, starchy vegetables like corn. Grains are another great source of complex carbohydrates, far less common in the United States, although we're making progress. (Or to quote a former roommate: "Grains? Aren't they for horses?")

Oh, Wilbur.

A SLICE OF CARBS

One of the easiest ways to eat more carbohydrates is to eat more breads—especially low-fat, whole-grain breads high in fiber. Bread suffered a bad rap for years as "fat food" and was usually the first thing to go in a diet. Today, it's rising to the occasion as one of the most healthful, convenient, and versatile foods on earth.

And maybe man can't live on bread alone—but I sure could! In fact, I love it so much I finally went out and bought a bread maker. Now I can make any kind of wholesome, non-fat bread my heart desires, and the hot, steaming results are so delicious that sometimes the loaf never makes it as far as the plate—which is why I have to periodically retire the bread maker to the top shelf of the cupboard to make sure I eat something else for a change. If you love bread as much as I do, I highly encourage you to splurge and buy one. That way you can guarantee that your bread is low or non-fat and high in fiber.

Meanwhile, let's put one myth to rest: There's no such thing as a bad bread; even balloon bread such as Wonder bread (the kind we wadded into a ball and threw at classmates in school, remember?) provides some fiber and nutrients, although whole-grain breads provide far more fiber and nutrients. (And forget trying to wad this bread into torpedo balls—it has too much fiber to scrunch down into a fistful.)

For "whole" goodness that delivers maximum fiber, check the label. You want to steer away from breads made with refined flour, where the germ and bran, as well as most of the nutrients, have been removed, including the Bs, Es, folic acid and minerals and fiber, and buy those whose first ingredient is either whole-grain or whole-wheat flour. (This wholeness principle, by the way, also applies to any products made with flour, including pancakes, waffles, crackers, etc.)

Some tips for buying the best bread:

1. Don't judge a bread by its cover. Ignore terms like "country," "rustic," and "multigrain" and go straight for the food label. If the first ingredient of the bread isn't whole-wheat flour or whole-grain flour, keep looking. Just because it says it's whole-grain doesn't mean it is.

2. Don't be fooled by "enriching" claims; all that does is add back a few B vitamins and iron without adding in any fiber.

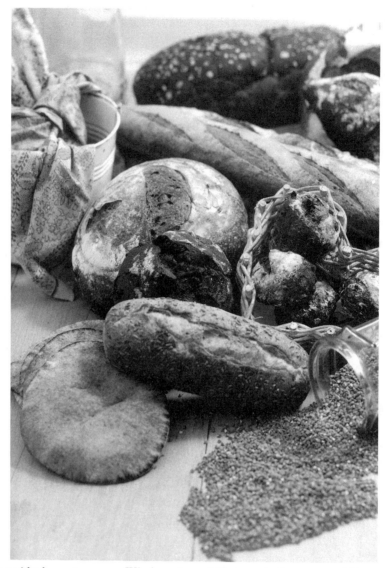

Bread is really an ideal energy source. Whole-grain varieties are a better source of fiber.

3. Choose low-fat breads. Most breads have no more than 2 grams of fat per slice so you're in luck here. Bagels, whole grain muffins, stoned-wheat crackers, whole grain crackers, and whole grain and dark breads are your best bet. Avoid croissants, buttery party breads, and pastries, and bakery-style muffins.

GRAIN PRIMER

Another way to up your intake of starches is to eat more grains, including corn, rice, oats, barley, and bran, and there are oodles of ways to eat them.

One easy way is to eat more breakfast cereal; today some whole-grain cereals offer 10 to 14 grams per serving or a half to a third of the daily RDA for fiber. For instance, Kellogg's All

Bran with Extra Fiber has 14 grams; General Mills Fiber One has 13 grams. Again, beware of imposters—just because a cereal says it's high grain doesn't mean beans. Look for cereals where whole-wheat, rolled oats, or whole-grain flour is listed first as the main ingredient and go with those that provide at least 4 grams of fiber.

Oatmeal, bran cereals, even some of the low-fat granolas are packed with whole goodness and little fat. Cooked grains are another way to go. Newer versions for fast-track cooks steam or microwave up in a jiffy and can be combined with steamed or raw vegetables for an instant nutritional feed.

Other grains that cook up fast and delicious are barley, which gives stews and soups a sort of chewy, rich texture and flavor or can be used as a base of casseroles and pilafs, or bulgur (it tastes better than it sounds). Use the dried or parboiled kind and you've got a nutritious meal in about 12 minutes. I love it toasted and tossed over salads or vegetables for a nutty flavor plus a fiber and protein boost.

Millet may sound like it's for the birds, but don't be fooled—it's great for people, too, and gives soups, stews, and pilafs a nutty flavor. Or toss a handful in your favorite bread recipe for instant crunch and nuttiness.

MARES AREN'T THE ONLY ONES WHO EAT OATS

By now everyone knows they should eat more oats. While not the miracle food manufacturers made it out to be, it's still a great source of nutrients and fiber. Try the new and improved oatmeals—no lumps! The minute-types let you boil up a breakfast in a jiffy, although even the old-fashioned versions are speedy and, in my opinion, taste a little better. Either way, oatmeal is a fiber-packed way to start your day, and it sticks to your ribs so you won't be tempted into mid-morning snacks at the vending machine. You can even toss some oatmeal into meat dishes and pilafs or add to stews as a non-fat thickener. If you really want to raise eyebrows, order porridge at a restaurant and enjoy it with non-fat milk and Equal for breakfast or a late-night snack. If you're in the South, grits are also a great grain—as long as you lay off the butter and gravy.

PASTA, PASTA

Finally, stock up on pasta and forget everything you've ever heard about them being fattening. One cup contains only 190 calories, less than a gram of fat, and no cholesterol. It's what you put on top that counts and counts, from greasy cheeses and meats to buttery sauces. Avoid them.

Try the new vegetable pastas—there's tomato, spinach, herb, even carrot pasta, to name a few.

For great, low-fat tips for cooking up a pasta storm, buy Norman Kolpas' *Pasta Light, 80 Low-Fat, Low-Calorie Fast & Fabulous Pasta Sauces,* (Chicago: Contemporary Books, 1991). From creamy spinach pesto to primavera with noodles, you'll learn which noodles go with what sauces, how to cook them up just right, and how to create low-fat sauces based on olive oil and herbs. Whether bucatini, linguine, vermicelli, or fettucine, you'll love it even if you can't pronounce it.

WISING UP TO FIBER

If you're like most Americans, you probably don't know beans about fiber. A 1992 study conducted by the National Cancer Institute found that only 18 percent of 22,000 adults surveyed knew that baked beans were a good source of fiber. And 20 percent listed white bread as a high-fiber food. Another 19 percent thought soda pop was high fiber! (It's not—unless you eat the cardboard carrier.)

Eat lots of carbs and you'll pretty much have the fiber part covered; the two naturally go hand in hand. Fiber is one of the most important contributions of a high-carb diet and comes in two forms: insoluble and soluble fibers. We need a little of both for maximum health. Insoluble fiber is found in wheat bran, whole grains, and vegetables. Insoluble fibers absorb water in the digestive tract, increase stool bulk, speed the movement of waste products through the digestive tract, and help prevent colon cancer, constipation, diverticulosis, irritable bowel syndrome, and hemorrhoids. They are the fibers that keep you regular.

Soluble fibers, such as vegetable gums and pectin, are found in fruits, oat bran, and cooked dried beans and peas. They have little effect on intestinal bulk and may even slow the movement of food through the digestive tract. But because they curb swings in blood-sugar levels and lower blood cholesterol, they help prevent or treat diabetes and cardiovascular disease.

Because fiber is filling and satisfying and has fewer calories, you can munch until your heart's content: eight cups of air-popped popcorn contain the same number of calories as one doughnut. High-fiber diets are also linked to weight management and a reduced risk of colon cancer and other major diseases. The National Cancer Institute, American Cancer Society, and American Heart Association recommend that Americans increase their fiber intake from current levels of approximately 10 grams a day to as much as 35 grams.

FIBER FIBBERS

Unfortunately, there are plenty of fiber imposters around. Some fiber bars and bakery goods and crackers range from nutritious to bogus and may be packed with fat, salt, and sugar. Read the label carefully; you may be buying more hype than high fiber.

Many that claim to be high-fiber, for instance breads with "bran," "wheat berry," "multigrain," or "cracked wheat" in the name, may have more white flour than any of those ingredients. That healthful brown appearance isn't the result of grains or wheat, but of caramel coloring.

A few fakers include rice cakes, Triscuits, couscous, any converted or refined rice products (Sorry, Uncle Ben), oatmeal cookies, or other junk food made with minimal amounts of grains.

While healthful in other ways, tofu is mighty lean on fiber. Ditto for celery, spinach, green peppers, pineapples, or grapes.

Here are a few foods that are packed with fiber, or contain at least 3 grams per serving:

- Whole-wheat spaghetti, buckwheat pancakes, popcorn, brown rice.
- Whole-grain cereals: Kellogg's All Bran with Extra Fiber, General Mills Fiber One, Wheat bran, Nabisco 100% Bran.
- Beans: in bean soups or casseroles using pinto, kidney beans, black-eyed peas, pork and beans and chili.

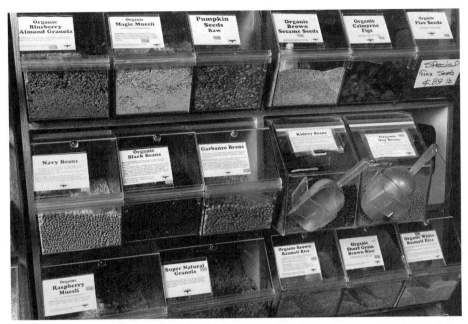

If you don't know beans about fiber, now's a good time to check out the grocery bins of your local supermarket. From pintos to chick peas, you can't go wrong. Even baked beans are better than no beans.

- Starchy vegetables: baked potatoes with skin, sweet potatoes, corn, and brussel sprouts all contain lots of fiber.
- Dried fruits: raisins, figs, prunes, and apricots. I always carry a box of raisins in my fanny pack for a low-fat, high-energy snack.
- Fresh fruit: apples, bananas, pears, etc.

To get your daily fiber, eat at least 5 servings of whole-grain breads and cereals, 4 servings of fresh fruits and vegetables, and a serving of cooked dried beans. Or try these tips to up your fiber intake:

1. Sprinkle oat bran into soups, stews, spaghetti sauce, meat loaf, hamburgers, or when you're making breads, muffins, waffles, or pancakes.
2. Use whole-grain cereals, such as Shredded Wheat, NutriGrain, or oatmeal.
3. Slice fresh fruit (bananas, strawberries) over your favorite high-fiber cereal.
4. Make sure your daily bread is 100 percent whole-wheat bread.
5. Think beans! They're loaded with fiber as well as protein and there are many types and ways to use them. Enjoy baked beans—they're not the villains you may think. Or add kidney, navy, pinto, garbanzo, or lima beans to salads, sandwiches, stews, and soups.
6. Munch on fresh fruit or vegetables—they're loaded with fiber.
7. Learn to cook with whole-grains such as rice, and use your noodles—whole-grain, of course.
8. Become a potato head. Baked potatoes are low in fat and packed with vitamins, minerals and protein—all for a skinny 150 calories per big potato.
9. Enjoy air-popped popcorn, a fun and low-fat way to eat lots of fiber.
10. For get up and go, drink prune juice. It's a proven remedy when things get sluggish.

THE RAW TRUTH ABOUT PROTEIN

While we all need some protein to repair bones, build and maintain muscle, grow hair and fingernails, and produce hormones and red blood cells, experts today recognize that it is weight-resistance training combined with protein and carbohydrate that builds muscle.

I agree with sports nutritionist Nancy Clark, R.D., that bodybuilders don't require any more protein than marathon runners or swimmers. In fact, a diet comprising about 15 percent protein and 60 percent carbs is an ideal diet for any athlete. However, some studies show that hardcore athletes, such as professional swimmers, weight lifters, or track stars, may need a little bit more protein than a couch potato, but it still falls within reasonable ranges.

Carbs are stored as energy in the muscles while protein doesn't provide fuel. If your muscles are lacking in carbohydrates, you simply won't have the energy you need to win the race or maintain the workouts required to build muscle.

Most of us eat enough protein without even trying. In fact, the average woman in the United States eats about 20 percent more protein than the Recommended Dietary Allowance (RDA) of 50 grams for women ages 25 to 50.

While meat and poultry are rich in all the B vitamins except folic acid, most of us aren't lacking in them, either, although eating enough iron and zinc on a meatless diet can be challenging, she adds.

Red meats are higher in iron, and poultry provides some, too. There are high levels of zinc in both red meat and poultry.

HOW MUCH IS ENOUGH?

If you're active, plan on eating at least a half a gram or more of protein per pound of body weight. To figure out how much protein you really need, divide your weight in pounds by two. For example, a 120-pound active woman would need at least 60 grams of protein per day (120 divided by 2). Considering that a 3-ounce serving of meat contains 21 grams, you can see that this doesn't entail stuffing ourselves with protein. In fact, eat a small can of tuna, a 4-ounce serving of meat, poultry or fish, trimmed or untrimmed, and you've already consumed about a third of your daily need.

Filling up on protein can actually cause vitamin deficiencies because you might be too full to eat enough carbohydrates. Also, protein breaks down into urea, a waste product which is eliminated in the urine. Too much protein can cause excessive urination, which may dehydrate you, or overtax your kidneys.

BEST SOURCES OF PROTEIN

Lean, skinless chicken, turkey, and fish are your best lean bets for protein, while pork, beef, and lamb are usually far more fatty. Don't assume that dark meat is healthier; in fact, dark meat is far more fatty than white meat. Throw in the skin and a serving of dark turkey meat or a piece of white chicken could contain more fat than a lean cut of beef.

For the leanest meat choice, stick to white meat without the skin and skip the wing, which is often considered white, but is actually fattier than the drumstick, even if you remove all the skin.

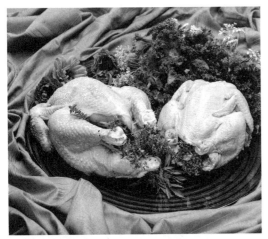

Chicken, turkey, and other types of poultry provide lots of protein with minimum fat (provided you eat it without the skin). Try it stuffed with fresh vegetables.

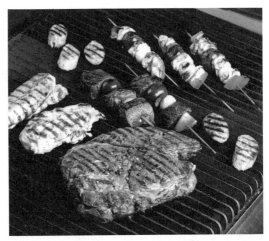

Shish kabobs are a tasty and low-fat way to grill chicken and fish, so fire up the barby!

Ground chicken and turkey can be a lean meal—but only if they're made from breast meat and no skin. Brands with poultry parts and skin can have five times as much fat as ground, skinless breast meat. Also, steer clear of products listing "turkey" or "chicken" as ingredients. That usually means the product contains meat plus fatty skin. Breast meat is the leanest.

When it comes to red meat, avoid ribs and porterhouse steaks, which are packed with fat. Instead, stick to round steaks, sirloin, top loin, and tenderloin. If a label doesn't list a grade, it could be anything, including the fattier choice, so go for round steak, whatever the grade, as well as top round, eye, bottom, and tip.

Finally, while light in color, pork isn't as lean as chicken or turkey. The usual cut has about a third more fat than skinless chicken and twice as much as turkey. And many of those lean figures apply only to tenderloin, which is very lean pork. I don't eat pork around my house—it really offends Beaver—and I wouldn't want to risk having his relatives for dinner.

Trimmed veal, on the other hand, has less fat than chicken.

PROTEIN PRIMER FOR VEGETARIANS

We all need some protein to build hair, bones, and repair muscle. Animal protein contains all 22 of these essential amino acids and is called a "complete" protein while vegetable protein is called "incomplete" because it lacks some of the amino acids.

You don't have to be a meat eater to consume all the essential amino acids, although if you're a vegetarian, you will have to pay a bit more attention to your diet. According to Clark, this entails learning how to combine certain foods for the same complete protein provided by meat. It's easy when you know how:

For breakfast: Milk and cereal or whole-grain toast bread

For lunch: Cheese and bread/pasta or pizza

For dinner: Grains, beans and legumes (rice and beans, tortillas and beans, corn bread and chili).

For snacks: Mix legumes and seeds; for instance, sesame seeds and chickpeas for a dip

STOCKING UP ON IRON AND ZINC

Plants are a poor source of iron, and the zinc in animal protein is absorbed 30 percent better than that in plants. Iron transports oxygen from the lungs to working muscles; without enough, you may become overly fatigued or even anemic. Zinc, which contains some 100 enzymes necessary for health, helps remove carbon monoxide from muscles during exercise and aids in healing. How to get your daily quota without eating meat? Either take supplements or stock up on foods high in one or the other. Since I'm basically a vegetarian and don't always eat a balanced diet the way I should, I take a supplement—just for insurance—to ensure adequate protein consumption.

To load up on zinc, eat oysters, tuna, lentils, or garbanzo beans. For iron, spoon up fortified breakfast cereals, grains and breads and slice strawberries on top to increase the absorption rate, or enjoy with a glass of orange juice.

Sprinkle wheat germ over cooked cereal for an instant iron boost or use cast-iron skillets for cooking and simmering sauces.

INTRACELLULAR WARFARE

But vitamins do more than fuel you nutritionally. Some even act as natural healers to protect your immune system from attack. In fact, one of the best ways to arm your immune system with a strong defense is to eat foods high in antioxidants—beta carotene, vitamin E, selenium, and vitamin C—vitamins that "gobble up" and envelop substances in the body called free radicals, which can cause pain and disease, explains Larrian Gillespie, M.D., a Beverly Hills urologist and founder and director of the American Foundation for Pain Research.

Let's take a look first at free radicals. Free radicals are inherently unstable molecules which have an odd number of electrons and react savagely with other compounds to cause pelvic pain. The ammonium ion in urine, for instance, is a very potent free radical. As they roam through tissue, they bind to and change the structure of cell membranes, making them more permeable so they leak. These reactive molecules obtain reactive oxygen from other compounds and often set off a chain reaction that creates yet other free radicals. The process continues indefinitely and is influenced from both within and outside of cells.

The normal use of oxygen by the body—or just breathing and being alive—can promote free radicals that cause molecular damage, or "insults" to cells. The number of these insults produced each day in each cell can run into the millions. These subatomic cracks or scratches in cells as well as in structures within cells, including genetic material, can disrupt a cell's normal work and actually impair its ability to protect itself from cancer and other diseases. For instance, free radicals can damage the tiny air spaces so that lungs fill with fluid. In the bladder, free radicals can attack the protective layer so the bladder becomes leaky. ("Honey, can we stop again? My free radicals are very active today.")

In addition to intracellular warfare, the formation of free radicals can be triggered by external factors outside the body, including heat, ultraviolet light, and other types of radiation, including X rays, cigarette smoke, alcohol (if you smoke or drink, here's another good reason to quit!) or such pollutants as nitrogen dioxide and ozone. Burns and other injuries can also lead to the formation of free radicals.

Not that free radicals are always bad or triggered by negative conditions. Even when no offending environmental factors are present, cells produce their own free radicals. White blood cells manufacture them as weapons against infectious bacteria and viruses. If genetic material damaged by free radicals is not repaired, the damaged DNA is replicated in new cells.

Living cells are not helpless in the face of free radicals. Just as cells can fight infection, the body can battle free radicals and repair molecular damage through systems that "swallow" or inactivate dangerous molecular by-products by sewing up the molecular holes, Gillespie explains.

MIGHTY ANTIOXIDANTS TO THE RESCUE

These free-radical fighters are called antioxidants. Some of these biochemical "good guys" are manufactured by the cells themselves. Others are actually nutrients that we eat. Whether the free radicals originated inside our body through intracellular warfare, or were caused by pollution or X rays, the right vitamins can "zap" them before they can cause damage.

While it's not quite understood how these free radicals cause diseases and disorders or how antioxidants gobble them up, researchers are increasingly convinced that a diet high in antioxidants promotes health and healing, according to Gillespie.

Maybe an apple a day won't keep the doctor away, but eating lots of broccoli, spinach, and oranges just might because these foods contain antioxidants which work together to boost your immune system and fight off infection. In addition, they may decrease your odds of developing immune-related disorders such as cancer by lowering cholesterol and cutting the risk of coronary disease. Since diet factors into 35 percent of all known cancers, it's important to eat your antioxidants—and every day. The way nutrition science is going, it may not be long before we go to a restaurant and order a "side" of antioxidants with breakfast.

GUIDE TO ZAPPERS

Among the most powerful antioxidants are vitamins C, E, beta carotene, or the substance in food that your body can convert to vitamin A, and selenium. Let's take a closer look at each one of these powerful free radical "zappers."

Vitamin C

Ascorbic acid, as it is also called, is water-soluble and found in all body fluids and may well be your first line of defense. A powerful antioxidant, it cannot be stored in the body and must be replaced regularly through fruits (like citrus fruits) and vegetables. Research shows that vitamin C may help reduce the risk of developing diseases that are associated with free radicals, such as cancer, heart disease, cataract formation, and birth defects.

Vitamin E

This fat-soluble vitamin is stored in the liver and other tissues. Scientists are currently studying vitamin E for its role in delaying aging, curing sunburn, reducing cataracts, preventing heart attacks, and gobbling up free radicals.

Beta Cartone (Vitamin A)

One of a large group of substances called carotenoids, which are generally found in dark green and yellow-orange vegetables and in fruits, beta carotene in the plants themselves protects them from solar radiation. In our bodies, carotenoids act as free-radical scavengers and may reduce the incidence of cataracts. Beta carotene also protects the skin and mucous linings of the nose—the body's first line of defense against attack.

Selenium

Selenium protects the cell walls from free radical damage and also strengthens the immune system's response to cancer growth.

BUILDING YOUR PERSONAL DEFENSE DEPARTMENT

Doctors generally agree that your best source of antioxidants is food—not supplements. Hoxter suggests that you make these power-packed foods a regular part of your diet.

High in Beta Carotene (Vitamin A:)

- Carrots
- Spinach
- Broccoli
- Winter Squash
- Tomatoes
- Melons
- Apricots
- Leafy greens

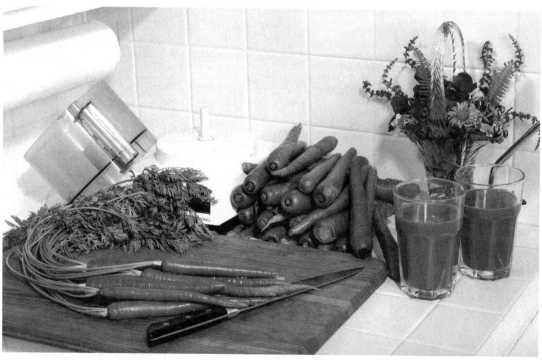

Bugs was right all along. But carrots are more than wonder food for wabbits. High in carotene, which is a potent antioxidant, they're a wonder food for people, too.

High in Vitamin C:

- Oranges, orange juice
- Strawberries
- Grapefruits/grapefruit juice

- Brussel sprouts
- Cauliflower
- Green peppers

High in Vitamin E:

- Sunflower seeds
- Safflower oil
- Almonds
- Peanuts
- Spinach

- Olives/olive oil
- Tomatoes
- Whole-wheat products
- Wheat germ

High in Selenium:

- Tuna
- Cod
- Chicken
- Noodles/spaghetti

- Cashews
- Skim milk
- Seafood
- Lean meats

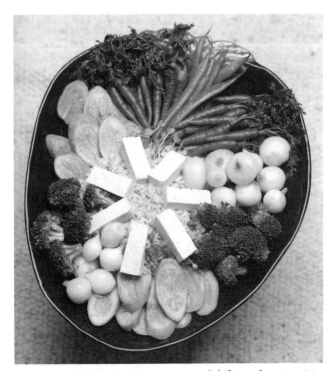

Turn this plateful of nutritious vegetables into your personal defense department.

THE HEALING POWER OF FOOD

Some diets are neutraceudicals—which means that they have healing powers or act like medicine. For instance, Gillespie has developed a special low-acid diet for her patients that actually "cools" the burning pain associated with cystitis.

And scientists have long known that a high-fat diet is linked to certain forms of cancer, including breast cancer; new research shows that diets high in antioxidants can significantly decrease the incidence of some types of cancer.

A new book called *Eat for Life: The Food and Nutrition Board's Guide to Reducing Your Risk of Chronic Diseases* (National Academy Press, Washington, D.C., 1993) offers a comprehensive explanation of how you can use food to boost your immune system and decrease your risk of the nation's top 12 diseases.

The Nutrition Board states that six of the 10 leading killers in America are directly related to diet—either too much of the wrong foods or not enough of the right ones. These include heart attack, cancer, stroke, diabetes, chronic liver disease, and atherosclerosis, while many others may result from a weakened immune system resulting from poor eating habits. A healthful diet may well speed recovery from surgery and illness and strengthen your immune system against infection. According to Darshan Kelly, Ph.D., of the USDA in San Francisco, even healthy people can suffer a lessening of immunity if their diets are inadequate—even if they look perfectly healthy. Unfortunately, a good diet is no guarantee; sometimes stress or genetics can wreak havoc on an immune system.

Doctors suggest that simple dietary changes could prevent 100,000 deaths each year in the U.S. In fact, in countries where the eating patterns approximate those suggested in *Eat for Life,* the mortality rates from diet-related cancers are less than half of what they are in the United States.

In addition to antioxidants, other vitamins and minerals can help you ward off infection, including vitamin B6, minerals such as iron, selenium, copper, and zinc—even garlic may have substances that inhibit the growth of bacteria and stimulate the immune system.

These same substances also greatly influence conditions in your mouth. Cosmetic dentist Dr. Steven Donia states that a diet high in anti-oxidants, vitamins, and minerals dramatically reduces gum disease (periodontitis) and associated tooth loss, and will help to keep you smiling with all the weight you lose with my book.

WHAT ABOUT VITAMIN PILLS?

More than 60 million Americans take them daily, but do we really need them? And at what levels do they do more harm than good?

The FDA can't ban vitamins—even if it considers a dose too high or so low that it's worthless. But it can prevent their vendors from making health claims.

Toxicities that accumulate over several months time are the biggest concern; another is that unlike prescription drugs or even meat, vitamins don't have to conform to a legal standard of purity. That vitamin pill you take may have 10 milligrams of a certain vitamin or 100, and you'd have no way of knowing.

Neither do they carry a list of side effects. To date, the U.S. government has no plan to remedy the situation. The law is that a harmful product can stay on the market until reports

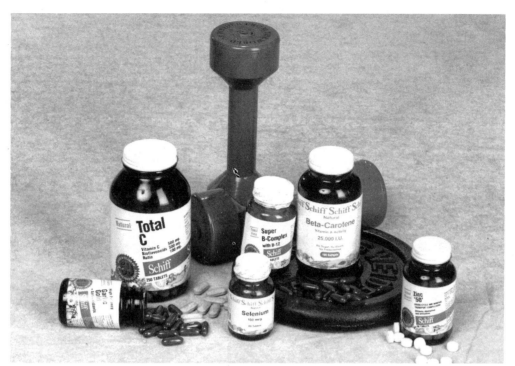

Should you take vitamins? Only your doctor knows for sure. Experts agree that, in general, it's better to eat vitamins rather than to swallow them in pill form.

reach the FDA. This may explain why an intravenous form of vitamin E which allegedly helped treat premature babies wasn't pulled off the shelves until 38 babies died and many more were injured.

For more information on vitamins, a helpful source is *The Right Doses: How to Take Vitamins and Minerals Safely,* by Patricia Hausman (Ballantine Books, New York, 1989).

A LOT TO DIGEST, HUH?

Still with us? I realize that this chapter was an awful lot to digest at one sitting—sort of like wolfing down Thanksgiving dinner in 10 minutes. Perhaps the best way to make these tips second-nature is to break this chapter and the next one down into minimeals and read a few sections every day.

Remember: the really great thing about our diet is that it's something we can control by simply keeping our mouths closed. So I'll make you a deal. If you improve your diet by cutting back on fat and increasing your intake of all the good guys, I'll quit my Snickers habit. Let's shake on it.

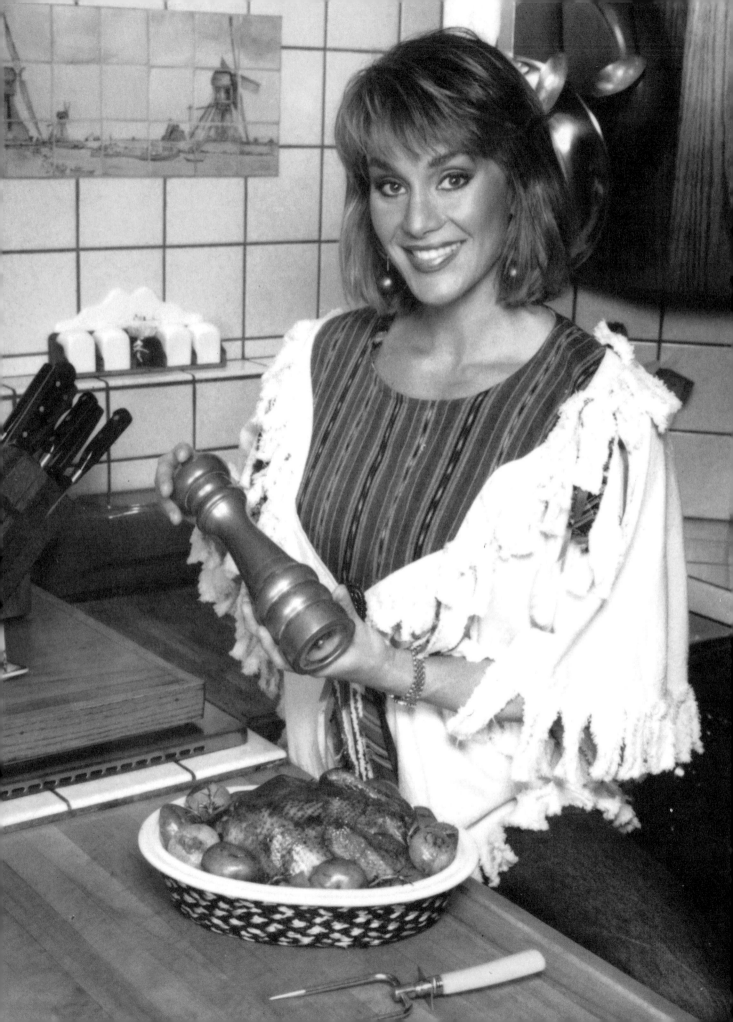

Five

Cory's Low-Fat Kitchen

Did somebody say eat MORE to weigh less? We sure did! It sounds like a paradox, but trust us: Diets are a fast route to weight gain and fat gain. Last year, Americans spent $32 billion on dieting. This year, statistics show that we're fatter than ever. And who needs statistics? All we really need are mirrors. Since it's clear that diets don't work, why not try something different for a change, like nondieting?

If you're ready to abandon calorie-counting, quasi-starvation, hunger pangs, and yo-yo diets once and for all, we can show you everything you need to know—from how to prepare a low-fat meal to slenderizing your favorite recipes, even your entire kitchen.

Your figure will love you for dropping the dieting. So will your metabolism. In fact, the only people who won't love you are envious friends who are still dieting—and growing fatter and fatter nibbling on lettuce leaves while *you* get thinner and thinner eating mounds of pasta—hold the butter, of course.

Repeat or yo-yo dieting not only drives your metabolism down to a snooze so you need less fuel to maintain the same weight but, as we discussed in Chapter 4, puts you at a higher risk of other medical problems because it's difficult to consume enough essential nutrients on a low-calorie diet. As we'll discuss more in Chapter 10, chronic dieting also makes you a sitting duck for eating disorders that are not only dangerous but sometimes deadly.

Finally, studies show that losing the same weight over and over again is actually more dangerous than not losing it all, according to Steven Blair, Ph.D., Director of Epidemiology at the Cooper Institute for Aerobics Research in Dallas. The more weight you lose, the greater your risk. Slim to moderately overweight people who maintain the same basic weight over the years have the lowest health risk.

Sometimes, not losing but gaining a few pounds as you grow older is the healthiest route, says Reubin Andres, M.D., Clinical Director of the National Institute on Aging at the National Institutes of Health in Baltimore. Studies show that those who are most likely to resist disease begin pencil-slim in high school and gain about a half a pound a year, which sounds good. Unfortunately, most of us weren't born looking like pencils.

The non-diet approach to weight loss revolves around feeding yourself real, delicious, low-fat food. No tricks or gimmicks.

FAST LOOK AT FAT

Let's take a look at fats first, the prime dietary villain, although, as we explained in Chapter 3, we all need some to survive.

Not all fats are created equal. Saturated fats, such as butter, margarine, and corn oil are the least healthy because they help boost cholesterol which can lead to heart disease, while monosaturated and polyunsaturated fats are more healthful because they tend to lower blood cholesterol, reducing heart disease.

A healthful diet gets 20 to a maximum of 30 percent of its calories from fat. Now think of your fat intake as a pie with three slices. One slice represents polyunsaturated fats such as corn or safflower oil, another slice is monosaturated fat, such as olive oil, and the last slice is saturated fat, such as butter, margarine, and oils found in salad dressings and many other products. Be careful, here, however. Even too much of the good oils can pad your hips and thighs with unwanted fat. Some of my friends and even famous chefs claim their lips never touch butter. Meanwhile, they consume enough olive oil to sink a ship! Good for cholesterol, bad for weight.

If you want to cut back on fat, the saturated category is the best place to do it. In fact, most people eat far too much saturated fat naturally in their diets without worrying about adding any.

The following chart shows the percentage of types of fatty acids found in common oils. Those with the highest amount of monounsaturated and polyunsaturated fats are most healthful and those with the most saturated fats are the least healthful. All of these pourable oils have 13 grams of fat per tablespoon and 120 calories.

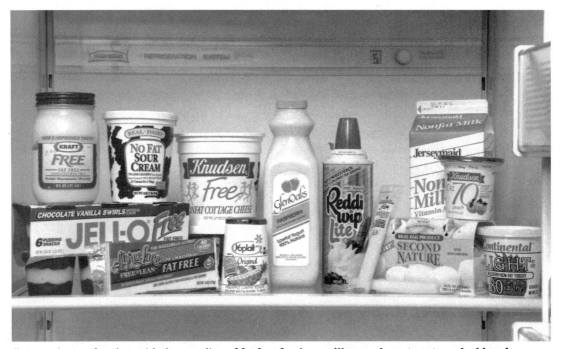

Fat may be our foe, but with the new line of fat-free foods, you'll never have to eat a naked lunch.

OILS	SATURATED	MONOUNSATURATED	POLYUNSATURATED
Canola	6	62	32
Safflower	9	13	78
Sunflower	11	20	69
Corn oil	13	25	62
Olive oil	14	77	9
Soybean oil	15	24	61
Cottonseed	27	19	54
Peanut	18	48	34
Salmon	20	55	55
Palm	51	39	10
Butterfat	66	30	4
Palm kernel	86	12	2
Coconut oil	92	6	2
Lard	41	47	12
Beef tallow	52	44	4

THE NEW WAVE OF LOW-FAT AND NON-FAT FOODS

Less than five years ago, low-fat foods were hard to find. You could find an odd can of this or that in the supermarket—and it was usually just that.

But if you wanted an entire low-fat meal, you were forced to flee to a spa or fat farm, where chefs did magic tricks in the kitchen, resulting in everything from low-fat strudel to non-fat chocolate cake.

Today, of course, supermarket shelves bulge with lean cuisine, some with less fat than a flea. Even bookstores have been fortified with low-fat information. So why aren't we getting thinner?

While non- and low-fat foods may be the easiest way to cut fat and be forever thin, that doesn't mean we don't crave the real thing—real butter on baked potatoes, for instance.

In an effort to satisfy our tastebuds while accommodating our desire for to lead a leaner lifestyle, manufacturers landed on what seemed a winning solution: They created a brave new line of fat-free substitutes to satisfy our cravings, gave them a taste and texture close enough to forgive the added or missing ingredients (fat, sodium, sugar, etc.), and they got fat (but did we get thinner?) on the profits.

Today, from sour cream wanna-be's to almost butter, there's a long list—growing daily—of non-fat substitutes faking it for the real thing. Unfortunately, many reduced or non-fat foods contain unhealthful amounts of preservatives, additives, and sodium to mask or compensate for taste.

While nutritionists agree that fat-free products are a legitimate way to reduce fat content, they also stress that taste should be your final judge. If you don't like the low- or non-fat substitute, don't force yourself to eat it just because it's lower in fat or you'll still crave the real thing and eat it too—and wind up consuming twice the calories. Trust me—I've done it.

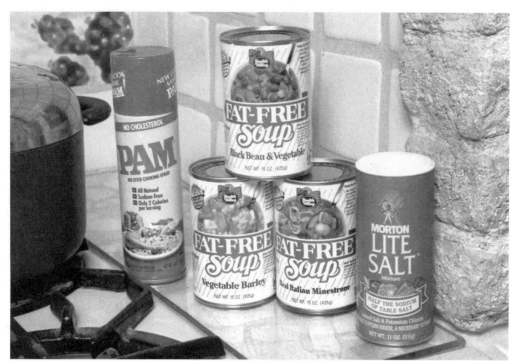

Non-fat snack foods such as fat-free popcorn, crackers, and cookies are giving high-fat counterparts a run for their money. Now there are no excuses.

THE SKINNY ON FAKE FATS

Are they safe—and really worth the calories they save? Or would we be better off just eating less real fat? Experts agree that while fake fats definitely save you fat and calories, studies show they are best used sparingly because those who abuse them tend to develop cravings for real fat and then binge, even if they didn't know the food they were eating contained fake fats.

Any of this sound familiar to you?

Nutritionists also fear that the advent of fake fats could encourage a new type of eating disorder: feasting on nutritional zeros—meals which have no fat, but no nutrients either. Meanwhile, the Center of Science in the Public Interest in Washington, D.C., a consumer advocate group, has asked the FDA to require that manufacturers of fake fats conduct studies to determine how they change the eating habits of those using them.

As of this writing, there are no fake fats suitable for cooking, baking, or frying, although Olestra by Procter & Gamble may be the first to obtain FDA approval. If and when it does, it's likely to appear in everything from cookies and potato chips to fried chicken.

Olestra (Procter & Gamble)

Olestra is nothing new. Procter & Gamble discovered it about 20 years ago while trying to come up with a formula for premature infants and wound up instead with a fake fat that could not be broken down by digestive enzymes.

The world rejoiced. Finally a free lunch! By replacing Olestra for fat in cookies, pies, deep-fried foods, and ice cream, we could pig out to our heart's content on all our favorite goodies without adding an ounce of fat.

It sounded too good to be true—and was. Further research showed that Olestra combined with fat-soluble vitamins such as A and E, thus removing them from the body. And in laboratory studies on rats, it caused leukemia, abnormal liver changes, and birth defects.

To date, research is ongoing and the jury is still out on Olestra. Because it has the ability to create a molecule that is foreign to the body, it may be harmful. On the other hand, it may prove to be totally safe, in which case it may one day revolutionize American grocery shelves.

Simplesse

A natural substitute fat, Simplesse is made from a protein blend of milk and/or eggs. Virtually cholesterol-free and containing just 1 ½ calories per gram, it has drastically slashed both the fat and calorie content of everything from ice cream and yogurt to chocolate chip cookies, pastries, salad dressing, spreads, dips, and margarine. Unlike Olestra, Simplesse breaks down during cooking and baking, limiting its use to frozen desserts and uncooked products. There are no known health risks for use in frozen desserts, although people who are allergic to eggs or milk products should avoid it.

Many people claim they actually prefer the "lite" versions of foods containing Simplesse to the real versions, while others can't stomach them and would rather splurge on the real thing less often than resort to a steady diet of fake fats. As for me, I can't tell the difference.

Wonderslim

A third, less known, fake fat is Wonderslim, a purée of dried plums and lecithin that is used to replace fat as well as eggs. A quarter cup contains 45 calories and may be used for a half cup of butter or three eggs—for a savings of more than 1,000 calories and 100 grams of fat. (Don't worry—Wonderslim won't have you racing to the nearest restroom the way too many plums and prunes could.)

DEMYSTIFYING CHOLESTEROL

This topic can really leave people scratching their heads so we're going to keep it very simple, because frankly, even scientists don't quite understand how it all works.

In a nutshell (where you won't find any, by the way) cholesterol is not fat, although it is a waxy, fatlike substance. It's found in all animals and animal products, including dairy products, meat, cheese, poultry—and humans.

The cholesterol we consume is called dietary cholesterol, to differentiate it from the cholesterol our bodies produce. Cholesterol is found both in the fat and lean part of meat but only in the fat of dairy products. Lean meat still has cholesterol, while skim milk and non-fat yogurt are essentially cholesterol free.

Unlike fat, cholesterol has no calories and supplies no energy. But it's no slouch that just sits in our bodies causing heart attacks, either. Cholesterol not only helps form cell membranes as well as the sheath that coats our nerves but is also essential for digestion and the production of hormones such as estrogen. Our body produces all the cholesterol it needs for these functions; in fact, usually far more than we consume from foods.

TWO TYPES OF CHOLESTEROL

There are two types of cholesterol: "bad cholesterol" or LDL (low-density lipoproteins) and "good cholesterol," or HDL (high-density lipoproteins). Both types are bundled with fat and protein, but LDL has more fat than protein while HDL has more protein than fat. (I know—it's very confusing.)

LDL, or bad cholesterol, can cause heart disease by clogging coronary arteries in people who have existing damage to arterial walls. No one is sure what causes this damage although theories include: virus infection; inherent weaknesses; diets too high in saturated fat. Tuck that last one away for a minute.

HDL, or good cholesterol, tends to protect against heart disease and may even carry cholesterol back to the liver for disposal or reuse, thus sweeping the arteries clean.

THE CHOLESTEROL-SATURATED FAT CONNECTION

Experts now believe that cholesterol and saturated fat are a deadly duo that work together to increase the risk of heart disease. In fact, studies of people in Mediterranean countries who eat diets very high in monosaturated fats (olive oil) also have extremely low rates of heart disease. Men who wake up to a glass of olive oil each morning live to be 100 years old. Why? Because their high-fat diet is low in saturated fat—the prime culprit.

But here things get confusing. Some people can live on French fries and hot fudge sundaes and live until 100; others would keel over and die by age 40.

When it comes to cholesterol, your genetic background is very important. To increase your odds of preventing heart disease triggered by too much fat in your diet, learn your cholesterol level.

Make an appointment with your doctor to get three things tested: your total cholesterol, HDL, and LDL. At least 25 percent of your total blood cholesterol should be HDL (exercise helps increase it, by the way.) The higher your HDL percentage, the lower your risk of heart attack.

If your total cholesterol count is high, you may need to carefully monitor your diet. A desirable range is less than 200 milligrams of cholesterol per 100 cc's of blood; borderline is 200–239, and high is more than 240. If your cholesterol level is 180 or lower and there is no history of heart disease in your family, you can probably get away with eating more saturated fat in your diet than if it's a risky 260, although I don't recommend it.

If you're sure you're doing everything right and you still have a high cholesterol count, remember that your genes may be a contributing factor. Ask your physician for some ways to cut your cholesterol and thus lower your total count. Or try a few of these tips.

HOW TO CUT CHOLESTEROL

- Cut back on saturated fat and you'll simultaneously cut back on cholesterol as well. Worst culprits include the sort of foods we stumble across in airports, at picnics, county fairs, and parties, such as greasy burgers, fries, cheeses, dairy products, butter, junk foods, hot dogs, sausage, etc.

- Read food labels for saturated fat and cholesterol counts.
- Load up on whole-grains and oats. Their high-fiber content helps lower blood cholesterol.
- Go fishing. Fish that live in cold oceans, such as salmon, mackerel, tuna, sardines, and herring offer natural protection against heart disease as well as hypertension, cancer, and arthritis. That's because the omega-3 fatty acids in these fish (a polyunsaturated fat found in fish oil) prevents the chemical reactions that cause blood to clot and which may exacerbate heart attacks. Forget fish oil supplements—they're expensive and pack far less omega-3 than the real thing.
- Eliminate cholesterol confusion by sending away for an entertaining video produced by two stand-up comics that tells you everything you ever wanted to know about cholesterol and saturated fat in a hilarious 35-minute tape. Called *Cholesterol Zone* ($22.95), you can get a copy by writing: Clever Cleaver Productions, 968 Emerald Street, Ste. 51, San Diego, CA 92109. The video comes with a booklet of 24, step-by-step recipes and basic information on preparing cholesterol-reduced meals.

YOUR PERSONAL FAT/CALORIE QUOTA

How much fat is enough? Studies show that those who eat less than 20 to 30 percent calories from fat often have diets lacking in vitamin B^{12}, niacin, and riboflavin. Your diet should contain no more than 30 percent calories from fat, preferably more like 20 percent if you're trying to lose weight. If you consume 2,000 calories a day, that's about 400 to 600 calories allowed from fat. A gram of fat has nine calories, so multiply grams of fat times 9 to see how many calories you're getting from them.

LOW-FAT COOKING 101

Perhaps the best way to lower the fat in your diet without feeling the pinch is to master the art of low-fat cooking. To give you a crash course, we asked Gayle Shockey Hoxter, M.P.H., R.D., nutrition expert for *Shape* magazine, to share the secrets she uses each month to transform high-fat meals into low-fat wonders.

Shockey says the changes may seem minor, but over the long haul they add up to make big differences in calories and fat. Just cutting one teaspoon of fat from your diet a day, for instance, can translate into more than four pounds a year.

FOUR BASICS OF LOW-FAT MAKEOVERS

1. Change just one ingredient at a time; e.g., reduce the fat or sugar content, or substitute non-fat for regular milk. That way if the recipe flops, you'll know what to blame it on.

2. Test the recipe first at home on your family—why flop in public or be a party pooper if you can use your hub and the kids as guinea pigs first? Besides, the kids won't lie as your friends might be tempted to do. A simple "yuck!" should cinch it. (Some of my meals are so bad that even Beaver turns up his snout.)

3. Start with teeny changes. Even if you only substitute out a little fat, it's better than none at all.

4. Keep your mouth shut—about the makeover, that is. It seems the minute people find out a dish is low-fat, they crinkle their noses and think dry cardboard. They're wrong.

Now let's look at how to make over your favorite home recipes, from baked goods to casseroles.

Desserts and Sweet Treats

Fat creates that rich, flaky texture we love in baked goods. But who needs the added calories and cholesterol?

- Substitute diet for regular margarine.
- Reduce the sugar in recipes and pump up the sweetness with spices such as cinnamon, nutmeg, or vanilla.
- Instead of using traditional pie crusts, which are packed with more than 50 percent calories from fat, use a low-fat graham cracker crust or filo dough, a low-fat Greek crust.
- Don't let the chips weigh you down in chocolate-chip cookie recipes. Halve the amount and you'll half the fat and calories.
- Use two egg whites for every whole egg. To increase tenderness and volume, beat the egg whites until they are stiff.

Main Courses

- Replace regular dairy products with low-fat or non-fat ones. Choose cheeses with less than 5 grams of fat per ounce.

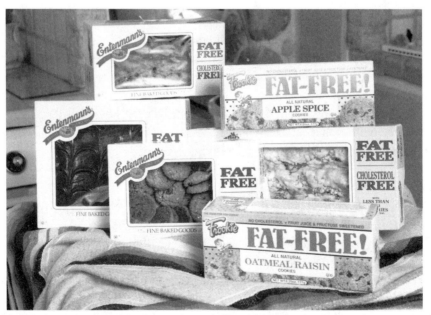

Low-fat goodies make it easier to get your sweet-tooth fix without turning into a plump sugar-plum fairy. Just remember to watch your portions: Non-fat doesn't mean no calories.

- Use tuna packed in water instead of oil and save about 180 calories per can.
- Use low-fat versions of cheese.
- Choose lean over fatty meats—turkey, chicken, lean beef, or 95 percent fat-free ham.
- Instead of cream soups, use chicken or beef broth or use the 95 percent fat-free cream soups.
- Thicken casseroles or soups with puréed rice or potatoes.

Side Dishes

- Sauté vegetables in wine or chicken broth instead of oil.

More Ways to Cut the Fat

Here's a grab bag of 35 more fat-savers from Hoxter.

- "Butter" toast with fruit-only jams instead of butter or margarine.
- Sauté meat and vegetables in chicken broth or wine; even if you don't drink, it's okay as the alcohol burns off during cooking.
- Use non-fat or low-fat dairy products; make your own rich skim milk by blenderizing it with a quarter cup of powdered dry milk per cup.
- Always remove skin from meat and poultry.
- Spread sandwiches with Grey Poupon mustard or low-calorie dressings and mayonnaise.
- To make low-fat tortillas chips, cut corn tortillas into triangles, bake until light-brown in the oven and enjoy with salsa, which has no fat and is low in calories.
- Take your own popcorn to the movies—the air-popped variety has half the calories and 0 grams (as opposed to about 15 grams) of fat per serving.
- Avoid cream soups, choosing broth-based soups or the newer, reduced-fat versions instead.
- Use evaporated skim milk in place of cream or half and half.
- Choose natural-style peanut butter, drain off the excess oil on the top for a savings of 130 calories and 14 grams of fat per tablespoon of fat drained off.
- Instead of basting or grilling meat with butter or oil, use vinegar, lemon juice, or defatted stock.
- Reheat leftovers in the microwave—you won't have to add any fat. Also, to reduce fat from ground beef, microwave it on a paper towel and toss the towel—and most of the fat, too. If your restaurant chicken looks greasy, dab it off with your napkin.
- Substitute water for about a third of the oil in any salad dressing, or try canned tomatoes, lemon juice, flavored vinegars, or non-fat yogurt.
- Cook up a batch of skinny lasagna, meat dishes, or stews by replacing about a fourth of the meat with cooked rice, ground turkey breast, or cooked oatmeal.
- Marinate raw meat in the fridge overnight or for about 12 hours and you won't even miss the fat you cut off to save calories.
- Some cows are fatter than others; Golden Trim, for instance, a brand of low-fat beef, is up to 98 percent fat free. The French Limousin cattle, which came to the U.S. in the 1970s, are more than 95 percent free of fat, with a top sirloin that weighs in with nearly a half of the fat as standard brands.

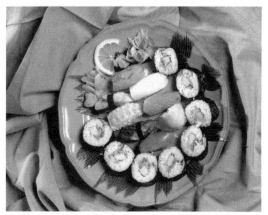

Sushi and vegetables—low-fat doesn't get any better. It's the most perfect meal in the world as far as I'm concerned.

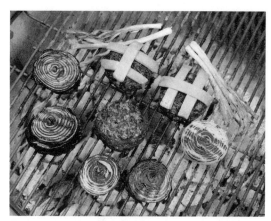

Cooking the low-fat way saves tons of calories, so grill rather than fry meat.

- Serve baked potatoes with low-fat cottage cheese, non-fat Ranch, or 1,000 Island dressing for a delicious and low-fat change of taste.
- Don't stuff your holiday bird with bread crumbs that soak up fat; instead, try seasoning it with citrus fruit and spices.
- Be a fat sleuth—learn how to read food labels and save foods with more than 3 grams of fat per serving for special occasions.
- Invest in a small fat counter—in a few months you'll automatically know which foods are fat monsters.

CREATING A SKINNY KITCHEN

One of the easiest ways to ensure low-fat cooking is to cut the fat from your shelves and restock them with low-fat substitutes.

Because it can be daunting (not to mention expensive) to toss out the bad stuff and restock your entire kitchen without professional assistance (some of you may also need a U-Haul), we asked Hoxter for some easy step-by-step tips to slenderize your total kitchen.

The Pantry

Don't buy any more of these.

Out: All oils except Canola, olive oil, and light brands; sugary, high-fat breakfast cereals; packaged or canned spaghetti, stews, or vegetables in sauce; beverages with sugar (soda pop, hot cocoa/hot chocolate mixes); creamed soups; junk food (fatty cookies, crackers, snacks, potato chips); olives; pasta and rice mixes with sauces; tuna and other canned meats and fishes in oil.

In: Canola and olive oil; whole-grain cereals and breads that are low-fat; fresh pasta, grains and rice; dried and canned beans; water-packed fish and meats; low-fat snacks and treats (the grocery shelves are crawling with them); and sugar-free beverages, coffee and tea.

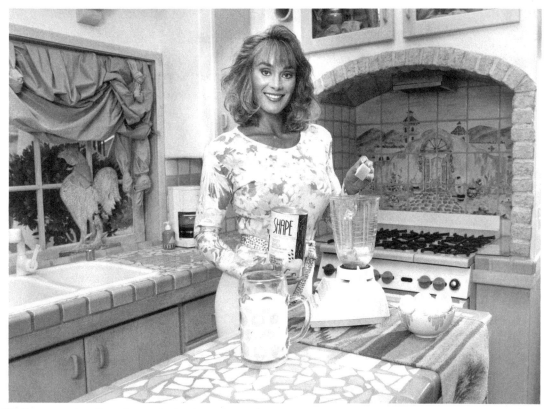

While competing, I used protein drinks and egg whites to supplement my diet. Remember, the yokes have all the fat.

The Fridge

Out: Butter and regular margarine; whole dairy products; eggs; high-fat meats, including many lunch meats; hot dogs; sausage; high-fat salad dressings and sauces; and regular yogurt.

In: Low or non-fat dairy products; low-fat salad dressings; lean cuts of meat; egg substitutes; fresh fruit; mustard; horseradish and pickles; lemon juice; non-fat sour cream and yogurt and non-fat dressings.

Stock your salad bin with salad greens and fresh vegetables—from asparagus to zucchini.

The Freezer

Out: Prepared foods that are breaded, prefried, or prepared in a sauce; creamed and buttered vegetables; fruit-juice concentrates with added sugar; regular baked goods and frozen dinners; high-fat desserts and pizza. Also, regular ice cream.

In: Lean meats and poultry (skinless); low-fat desserts and ice cream; frozen vegetables without sauces; low-fat frozen entrées; berries. Also stock up on whole-grain bagels, breads, rice cakes, pita breads, and English muffins.

Note: Don't freeze mayonnaise, yogurt, milk, cheese, eggs, fruits and vegetables with high water content, like cucumbers or lettuce, or foods whose labels warn against refreezing after thawing.

Freezer Life

To ensure freezer-friendly foods, label and date freezer containers, arranging the oldest stuff in the front of your freezer. Grocery-packed meats, turkey bacon and sausages will last about two months in the freezer; sauces, low-fat puddings, about three months; fresh herbs, about four months; fruits, vegetables, breads and baked desserts, about six months; pasta, potato dishes and casseroles, about 10 months; and raw meat, poultry, fish, dried herbs and spices, about a year.

Produce Bin

Out: toss (or give to the neighbors) avocados, olives, nuts and high-fat seeds.

In: fresh fruits, vegetables, garlic, onions, potatoes (sweet and Russet), yams.

Condiments

Reducing the fat, sugar, and salt content of your favorite foods can lead to lackluster results, which is where healthful condiments and spices come in. By learning how to use them to fill flavor voids, no one but you will ever know what's missing.

Out: High-fat gravy and sauce mixes; salty or high-fat condiments, such as mayonnaise, soy sauce, ketchup, Worcestershire sauce, and bouillion cubes.

In: Garlic powder; light salt; pepper; reduced-sodium sauces and condiments; salt-free seasonings; salsa and Tabasco; low- or non-fat sauces and dressings; a variety of spices, including basil, bay leaves, oregano, and herb spices for cooking; butter flavoring, ginger, nutmeg, and cinnamon and vanilla, orange, and other extracts for baking.

Note: Spices retain their flavor best when stored whole in a cool place, rather than ground and packaged. Most commercial spices last six months on the shelf, or a year in the freezer.

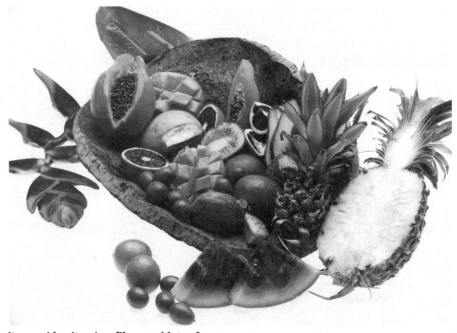

Fresh fruits provide vitamins, fiber, and lots of energy.

Lean Machines

In addition to having the right food around, you also need the right tools. Here are a few fat-slashing gadgets for creating a streamlined kitchen.

- Containers, ice-cube trays, and plastic freezer bags: For storing leftovers into single-portion eating. Freeze liquid seasonings and stocks in ice-cube trays and drop cubes into soups and stews for instant flavor.
- Double meat loaf pan: Fitted with a perforated inset so fat drips into an outer pan.
- Portable hibachi or a simple grill: Gives foods a smoky richness. Invest in a few skewers for low-fat meals in a flash.
- Nonstick skillet: The most important pan in your kitchen, use it to bake, fry, sauté, and even boil foods. Use a squirt of non-stick cooking spray and nothing will stick. Buy one that is 12 inches in diameter and 3 inches deep with a fitted lid and oven-proof handle. Use plastic or wooden utensils to avoid scratching the non-stick surface when preparing food.
- Parchment paper: Low-fat cooking containers to hold marinated beef and vegetables.
- A chef's knife and a paring knife: For slicing meat and vegetables paper thin, and removing all the visible fat from poultry and meats. Combination carbon/stainless steel knives are best.
- Strainers: Steel or plastic versions trap fat that would otherwise go into your food.
- Fat separators: For skimming fat from hot liquids.
- Blender: For whirring up smoothies, soups, bisques, spreads, dips, and desserts. The new hand-held immersion blenders are easy to use and clean.
- Food scale: Eliminate guesswork and helps you learn to eyeball correct amounts. The flat, rectangular food scales are more stable than older, postal-scale models.
- Spice grinder (or small coffee grinder): Spices lose their punch after sitting around on a shelf for months and we rarely use them up fast enough. With a grinder you can purchase small amounts of whole spices and grind them on the spot to enjoy their full flavors.
- Steamer: Protects against nutrient loss and cooks vegetables without grease. The double and triple-decker varieties let you steam several different foods at once.
- Wok: For stir-frying in a low-fat way to make quick, delicious meals with minimum oil. A necessity for creating low-fat Chinese fare. If you don't want to invest in a wok (about $10), you can use a large frying pan. Fresh vegetables done stir-fry are wonderfully crunchy and crisp and keep their nutritional value lost by boiling.
- Yogurt cheese funnel: If you're a yogurt fanatic, you can make your own with this helpful little gadget that eliminates the mess and fuss of using cheesecloth.
- Microwave oven: You probably already have one (I would starve without mine). If not, what are you waiting for? With a microwave oven you can cook up foods lickety-split with minimum fat and also take advantage of the new line of low-fat microwavable meals. And where would a modern-day girl be without microwave popcorn? Pop it up and take a bag with you to the movies for a low-fat crunch.
- Hot-air popcorn popper: These pop up a bowlful without any fat or oil and eliminate scorched kernels.
- Broiling racks: If you have a standard oven, you probably already have one. If not, invest in a few. Broiling is a non-fat way of cooking meat, fish, potatoes, and veggies which adds a rich flavor.

BRAVE NEW FOOD LABELS

Another way to cut fat is to learn how to read food labels. You'll be amazed at the differences between similar products when it comes to fat content. Unfortunately, until lately, the labels were so confusing and often so misleading that they were hardly worth the paper they were printed on.

For instance, many cereals claim to be high fiber or "whole grain" but aren't, or you buy "fruit" juice only to find that there was more fizz than real fruit. Don't get me started on "lite" desserts which are only "lite" in terms of the serving size—obviously sized for Lilliputians or mice. But my favorite scams are those "cholesterol-free!" peanut butters, even though peanut butter has never contained cholesterol because cholesterol is animal fat and peanuts are vegetables. (Remember, peanut butter does contain a lot of fat.)

But hope is on the way—and soon. By 1994, food labeling hype will pretty much be boxtop history. The federal government has come out with new food labeling laws that will not only cut to the nutritional chase but make it pretty hard for manufacturers to fudge the nutritional facts.

Not only will the new labels tell us exactly how much saturated fat, cholesterol, dietary fiber, and other nutrients we're eating per serving but what's healthy about the particular product. So long, "cholesterol-free" peanut butter!

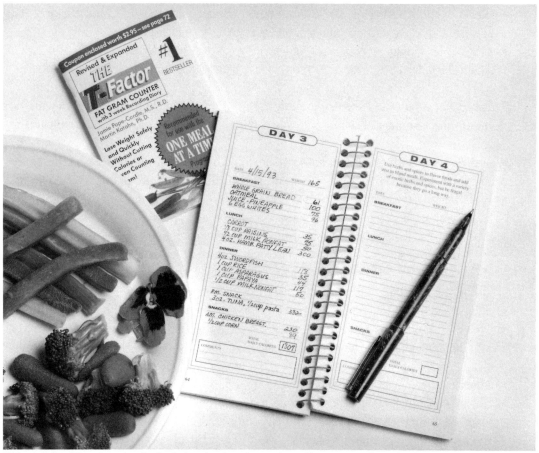

Keep track of fat grams and caloric intake, in a journal, until your new diet plan becomes habit.

LOW-FAT MEAL PLANS

Whether you're a certified grazer, lover of gourmet cuisine, or a vegetarian, there's a low-fat meal plan to suit your taste buds. Below is a 7-day meal plan from Gayle Shockey Hoxter, M.P.H., R.D., followed by six one-day plans. Feel free to mix and match them for 42 different meal plans in all averaging between 1,500 and 1,800 calories, with options for higher-calorie meals.

1. Shockey's Seven-day Shape-up

Snacks: (pick two per day and enjoy when hunger strikes!)
4 graham crackers,
1 cup non-fat yogurt or ice milk

1 piece fresh fruit
Bagel with low-fat cream cheese
4 cups air-popped popcorn

DAY 1

Breakfast:
1 cup bran flakes with 1 cup sliced strawberries
1 cup skim milk

Coffee or tea

Lunch:
Turkey sandwich (two slices whole-wheat bread, 2 oz. turkey, 1 tbs. diet mayonnaise or mustard, lettuce, tomato, and sprouts)

1 cup low-fat fruit yogurt
5 vanilla wafers
Low-calorie beverage

Dinner:
Pasta Salad (1 ½ cups cooked pasta, 1 cup broccoli florets, ¼ cup red pepper, diced tomato, 2 oz. cubed mozzarella, 2 tbs. fat-free dressing)

1 slice Italian bread with 1 tsp. diet margarine.
Low-calorie beverage

DAY 2

Breakfast:
1 cup cooked oatmeal with cinnamon
⅓ cup unsweetened applesauce
2 tbs. raisins

1 cup skim milk
1 orange
Coffee or tea

Lunch:
Spinach salad (1 cup fresh spinach, 1 cup hard chopped egg, ⅓ cup chick peas, ¼ cup mushrooms, onions, sprouts, 4 cherry tomatoes)

8-inch pita pocket
Peach
1 cup frozen yogurt
Low-calorie beverage

Dinner:

3 oz. barbecued chicken

Fresh vegetable sticks

Small muffin with 1 tsp. diet margarine

1 cup fruit

½ cup small salad with fat-free dressing

Low-calorie beverage

DAY 3

Breakfast:

½ cup non-fat cottage cheese with ½ cup
    fresh fruit

Small bran muffin with 1 tsp. low-calorie fruit
    preserves

Coffee or tea

Lunch:

2 slices vegetarian pizza with low-fat cheese,
    mushrooms, pineapple chunks, peppers

1 cup salad with 1 tsp. fat-free dressing

Low-calorie beverage

½ cup ice milk

Dinner:

4 oz. broiled fish

1 cup red potatoes

1 cup cauliflower

1 roll with 1 tsp. diet margarine

1 cup fat-free frozen yogurt

Low-calorie beverage

DAY 4

Breakfast:

Soft-cooked egg

1 slice whole-wheat toast

1 cup fruit

Coffee or tea

Lunch:

Tuna pita sandwich (2 oz. water packed tuna,
    ⅓ cup sprouts, ⅓ cup diced tomato,
    cucumber, 1 tbs. fat-free mayonnaise)

3 fig newtons

1 cup skim milkshake (made with low-fat ice
    cream or non-fat dairy dessert)

Dinner:

4 oz. lean tenderloin

1 cup steamed zucchini with 1 tbs. Parmesan
    cheese

Baked potato with 1 tbs. sour cream substi-
    tute

Dinner roll with 1 tsp. diet margarine

Low-calorie beverage

DAY 5

Breakfast:

2 frozen waffles with 2 tbs. low-calorie syrup

1 cup fresh or frozen fruit

Coffee or tea

Lunch:

Chef Salad (1 oz. lean chicken, 1 oz. lean ham, 2 oz. low-fat cheese, 1 cup lettuce, sprouts, tomatoes, cucumbers, onions, etc., with 1 tbs. fat-free dressing)

1 whole-wheat roll
1 cup non-fat fruit yogurt
Low-calorie beverage

Dinner:

3 oz. Cornish hen
½ cup rice pilaf
1 cup broccoli/carrots

1 cup sliced tomatoes
1 slice angel food cake with ½ cup fresh fruit
low-calorie beverage

DAY 6

Breakfast:

Strawberry-banana yogurt shake (¾ cup non-fat plain yogurt with 1 banana and ⅔ cup fresh or frozen strawberries and 2 to 3 drops vanilla extract)

1 slice whole-wheat toast with 2 tsp. low-calorie jam or preserves

Lunch:

Baked potato with ½ cup spinach, ¼ cup non-fat cheese, ¼ cup mushrooms and 1 tsp. Parmesan cheese

1 cup non-fat yogurt with ½ cup fresh fruit
Low-calorie beverage

Dinner:

1 cup whole-wheat pasta with ½ cup low-fat tomato sauce
1 cup mixed salad with 1 tbs. fat-free dressing

Roll with 1 tsp. diet margarine
1 slice fat-free cake with ½ cup non-fat ice milk

DAY 7

Breakfast:

2 whole-wheat pancakes with ½ cup strawberries
1 cup orange juice

1 cup skim milk
Coffee or tea

Lunch:

Skinny Spanish omelet (2 egg whites scrambled with ½ cup fat-free refried beans, 2 oz. fat-free cheese, fat-free sour cream, ¼ cup salsa)

1 ½ cup green salad with 1 tbs. fat-free dressing
1 cup non-fat yogurt

Dinner:

3 oz. broiled chicken
1 cup mashed potatoes (made with non-fat milk and diet margarine)

Small muffin with 1 tsp. diet margarine
1 cup fresh fruit
Low-calorie beverage

2. Cory's Favorite Foods Diet
I'd eat this every day if I could! In fact, just thinking about it makes my mouth water.

Breakfast:
1 bagel with 1 tsp. non-fat cream cheese   Coffee with non-fat milk.
1 cup fresh berries

Midmorning snack:
Cinnamon rice cakes

Lunch:
Two slices veggie pizza (hold the cheese)   1 cup non-fat milk
1 cup spritzer

Mid-afternoon snack:
4 cups airpopped popcorn

Dinner:
3 oz. broiled fish or sushi   1 cup green salad
½ cup pasta with vegetables   1 cup low-fat milk.

Evening snack:
Non-fat frozen yogurt, or a handful of jelly
    beans, or animal crackers or, if I've
    earned it, a miniature (2.16 oz.) Snickers
    bar.

3. The Grazer Diet
Perfect for those who prefer several mini-meals to three large ones.

Breakfast:
1 cup oatmeal or cooked cereal with low-fat   1 slice whole wheat toast with 1 tsp. diet mar-
    milk and one teaspoon sugar   garine
    1 glass orange juice

Midmorning snack:
1 cup fresh fruit

Lunch:
Turkey sandwich on whole-wheat bread with   1 cup tossed salad with 2 tsp. non-fat dressing
    1 tsp. Grey Poupon   Low-calorie beverage

Mid-afternoon snack
1 cup non-fat yogurt

Dinner

4 oz. broiled fish

Baked potato with non-fat sour cream and
  chives

½ cup steamed vegetables

1 cup low-fat milk

Low-calorie beverage

Evening snack:

4 cups air-popped popcorn

4. Flash Diet For those in a hurry.

Breakfast:

Bagel with 1 tsp. non-fat cream cheese and
  sugarless jam

Apple or orange

Coffee or tea

Mid-morning snack:

Orange

Lunch:

½ can water-packed tuna mixed with cottage
  cheese and spread on stone-wheat crackers
  or bread

1 cup non-fat milk

Banana

Mid-afternoon snack:

6 low-fat crackers such as Matzo

Dinner:

1 cup meatless chili

1 slice cornbread with 1 tsp. diet margarine

1 cup green salad with 1 tbs. fat-free dressing

1 serving non-fat dessert or frozen yogurt

5. Exercise-Lovers Diet
For those who love to aerobicize, this diet will provide the power you need to keep
moving.

Breakfast:

1 large banana sliced over 1 cup bran flakes

1 cup non-fat milk

Coffee or tea

Lunch:

Branola bread veggie sandwich with low-fat
  cheese

Orange

Low-calorie beverage

Snack:

4 non-fat cookies

Dinner:

3 oz. broiled fish
Corn on the cob with 1 tbs. diet margarine
½ cup broccoli

1 cup non-fat frozen yogurt
Low-calorie beverage

6. Skinny Gourmet Diet
For those who love gourmet cuisine minus the calories and fat.

Breakfast:

Half baked grapefruit with 1 tsp. sugarless
    preserves
2 whole-grain pancakes topped with strawber-
    ries and ½ cup non-fat vanilla yogurt or
    lite syrup)

Coffee or tea

Lunch:

1 cup seafood pasta salad with fat-free com-
    mercial dressing

1 cup fresh fruit sorbet
Low-calorie beverage

Dinner:

3 oz. broiled salmon
½ cup steamed asparagus
Whole-grain dinner roll

1 cup non-fat ice milk parfait (ice milk layered
    with fresh fruit and a strawberry on the
    top)
Low-calorie beverage

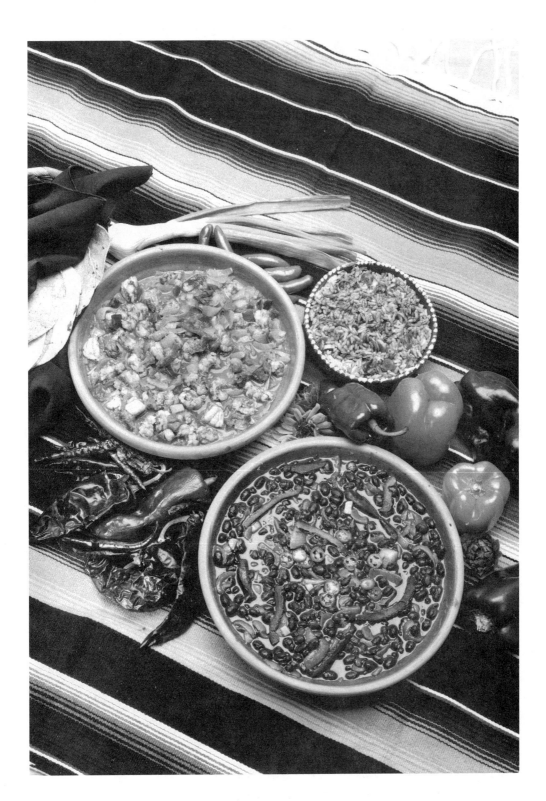

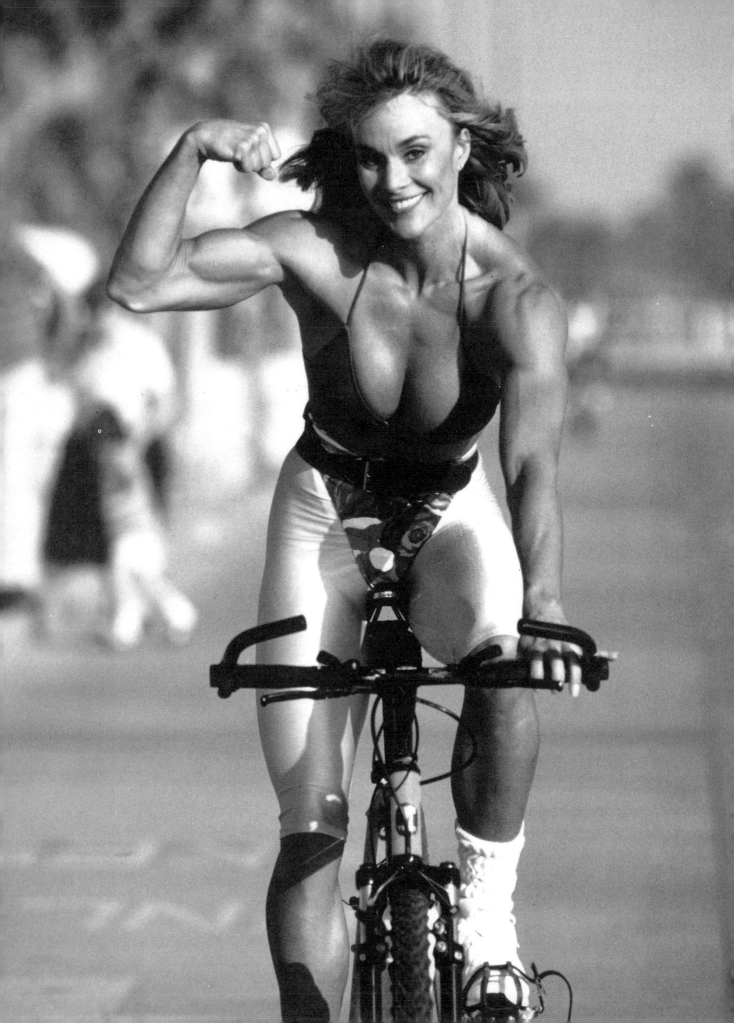

Six

Move It to Lose It

Want to maintain your ideal weight for the rest of your life—and never diet again?

Eating nutritious, low-fat meals is half the solution. But to keep flab from creeping back like the Blob, you'll also need a regular exercise program. Or, as the saying goes, you have to move it to lose it.

Don't panic! We're talking less than four hours a week here, girls, less time than most of us spend on our hair and nails and they're DEAD cells. Don't our living bodies deserve the same attention and consideration? So that old "so little time" excuse won't hold water. If you have time to pick up a blow dryer, you have time to pick up a dumbbell. And if you're still convinced after reading this chapter that you just can't squeeze exercise into your life, send me your weekly calendar. I'll find room for it!

Spending those four hours working out will make a bigger difference in the quality of your life than anything else you could possibly do with them. In fact, they can be the difference between a lifetime of battling fat and the satisfaction of maintaining your weight with minimum sweat.

WHEN FAT HAS A FIT

According to Philip Walker, M.S., fitness management consultant for the Cooper Clinic in Dallas, Texas, the folks who made aerobics a household term, there's another hidden benefit to getting in shape. As your fitness level increases, your physiology shifts so that your body burns more fat no matter what you're doing. Most overweight people don't eat more—they just burn less fat. To put it another way, the more fit you become, the more your body naturally resists fat.

I know that probably sounds too good to be true, but take it from me. If someone had tried to tell me when I was a professional bodybuilder that I only needed to work out four hours a week to stay in shape as opposed to the four to six hours a day I was enduring, I would have told them to go fly a kite. But it turned out to be true.

When I left professional bodybuilding in 1989, my available workout time dropped from six hours a day to less than four hours a week. Adios muscles, I said to myself, secretly wondering if I'd have a battle to keep from resembling Mr. Beaver, my 250-pound, pot-bellied pig.

I can't tell you how astonished I was to discover how little workout time it really took to maintain my muscle tone and low body fat. Would you believe 30 minutes of weight training three times a week and another 30 minutes of aerobics four times a week?

That's a grand total of three and a half hours a week—or less time than I used to work out every single day!

Exercise experts had been saying this for years, but I didn't believe it until I had personal proof. Once you achieve a level of fitness that's ideal for you and maintain it for at least six months, your body develops what's called "muscle memory" and not only remembers how to stay in shape but actually resists getting out of it. Even missing a few workouts or pigging out on brownies once in a while won't hurt—you'll really have to work to get out of shape. Take it from someone who truly put this theory to the test.

WHO ME, EXERCISE?

If you qualify for couch-potato status, you may be tempted to bolt at the very mention of the "E" word, if you have the energy to do so. Which brings up another hidden bonus of exercise—the sheer energy it gives you—not only for your workouts but for every single thing you do in life.

HI-HO, HI-HO

Show me a successful woman and I'll bet you ten to one that when she ends her day at the office, she kicks off her heels, laces up her Nikes and hi-ho, hi-ho, it's off to the gym she goes to recharge her physical and mental batteries. Fitness and success go hand in hand.

Exercise doesn't have to be torture, and it doesn't have to leave you gasping for air. Once you develop the habit, nothing will get in your way; it becomes as natural as eating and sleeping. I could have twelve phone messages waiting for me on my answering machine, but if I'm raring to speedwalk, a call from Kevin Costner couldn't stop me from rushing out the door—Sorry, Kev.

THE MIGHTY TRIO

Getting fit isn't a big deal—or even a fulltime job. In fact, once you commit to the program (which is often the hardest part) it's as easy as one, two, three: Stretching, Aerobics, and Weight Training.

- Stretching improves flexibility, posture, and body awareness, leading you in the right direction to an active, injury-free lifestyle.
- Aerobics builds stamina and endurance by increasing your cardiovascular capacity, or wind.

- Weight training strengthens and tones your muscles for strength and builds a more shapely and symmetrical body, so you wind up with the best version of you.

But why three different types of exercise? Wouldn't just one do the trick? In a word, no.

Walker often sees professional athletes at the Cooper Clinic who are anaerobically fit (muscle bound) but wheezing geezers when it comes to aerobics.

Not long ago, a professional sprinter dropped by the clinic to test her aerobic capacity. Her big race was the next day and she was in prime form—anaerobically speaking, that is. But when Walker put her on a treadmill, within 15 minutes she was totally pooped. What was going on here?

Her training, which involved sprints less than a minute long, didn't build the endurance needed for longer hauls. The woman went on to win her sprint the next day and Walker wasn't surprised, as this was exactly what she had trained for. But had that sprint been a 3-mile run, she might have come in last.

I've known many amateur and professional bodybuilders who fall into the half-fit category. They have well-developed muscles but no wind. I have a close friend who can pick up and move my piano. But ask him to go walking and he's gasping for breath before we make it around the block.

There's a saying that you get what you train for and if you don't train right, you really get it! The wonderful thing about a three-in-one exercise program is that it does it all. Stretching keeps you flexible and able to make the moves your sport requires without risking soreness or injury. Aerobics burns body fat and increases your endurance, giving you everlasting energy, while weight training takes up where aerobics leaves off, making you even stronger and more shapely than ever.

Leave out just one component and you end up with half or a third of your fitness potential—even if you spend twice the time on one form of exercise that you would spend on all three a week.

If you want to look like a champ, train like one. The pros are far too busy to waste time.

One caveat: If you're more than 20 pounds overweight or recuperating from a serious illness or injury, check first with your physician before starting this or any new exercise program. Now let's get started.

STEP ONE: STRETCHING

Okay, so stretching is not a thrill a minute. In fact, if you're like me, you'd rather scrub the toilet or clean the birdcage. But while stretching before and after workouts may be a yawn, skip it and soon you'll wish you hadn't.

According to National aerobics champion Michelle LeMay, most people are not aware of the many benefits of stretching, which is why it's often the forgotten element of fitness. First of all, even if you never worked out a single day in your life, chances are you would still have muscle tightness and tension from stress. Stretching warm muscles is probably the most effective way of reducing muscle tightness, tension, and stress. In addition, it promotes mental clarity, allowing you to experience mental relaxation.

Stretching complements muscular strength and development and allows for greater physical gain. The more flexible you become, the more effective your muscles work, and in turn you experience an increase in coordination and agility.

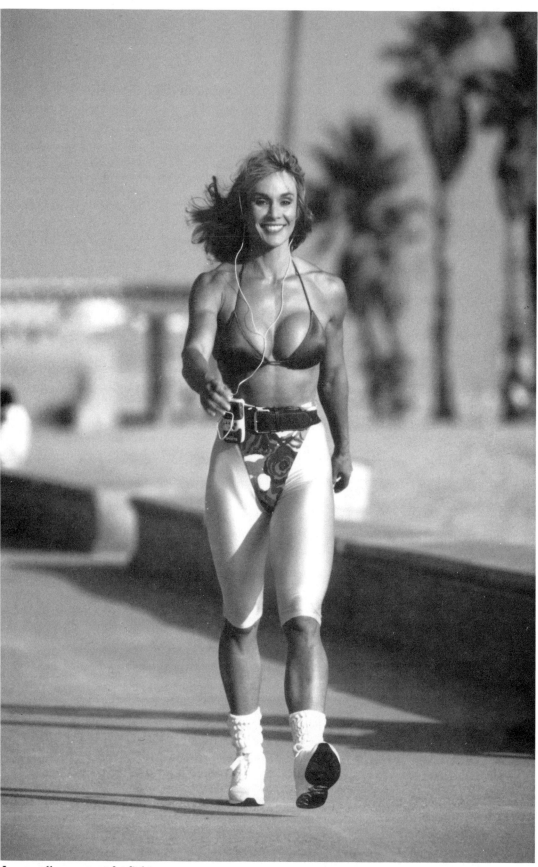

Long walks are great fat fighters.

Convinced to stretch yet? If not, let me enlighten you with a few more benefits. Stretching makes you feel good, improves posture, enhances your overall body awareness and, on a medical note, improves circulation. Lastly, something near and dear to me, due to a recent experience: Stretching reduces the risk of muscle soreness and injury!

I recently finished a role in a movie in which I play a martial arts fighter. I memorized every line, but neglected to do any stretching. After two days of high kicks, jumps, and leaps, I knew the true meaning of sore. I hobbled around the house like a little old lady smelling like Ben Gay. So don't think it can't happen to you. Even us know-it-all professional athletes need to take a bit of our own medicine. So make stretching a part of your workout, using light stretching before workouts and saving deep stretching for after workouts, when your muscles are warm and limber.

STEP TWO: AEROBICS

The greatest fat-fighter of all activities! While many forms of exercise burn calories, aerobics is the only form of exercise that actually burns body fat while exercising. Ever wonder why aerobic instructors seem to run around with endless energy all the time? Michelle LeMay says, "Aerobics crank up your metabolism for up to 15 hours after your workout, giving you energy galore and ready for more." Think of it as a victorious cycle! The more fit you get, the easier it is to stay that way.

Aerobic exercise is any type of activity that has you working within your target heart rate range continuously for at least 20 minutes and that forces your body to use large amounts of oxygen. This makes your body better at transporting life-sustaining oxygen to all your cells.

Aerobic activities which use the large muscles of the hips and thighs burn the most calories; however, it's still a matter of what you put into it. As I said earlier, the best exercise for you is the one that you enjoy the most. Cycling, walking, jogging, hiking, cross-country skiing, in-line skating, and mountain biking are fabulous outdoor fat-fighters. Aerobics classes and exercise machines such as treadmills, exercise cycles, and stair climbers are some excellent ways to ditch the fat indoors.

Don't let the sweat from sports such as tennis, racquetball, and squash fool you into thinking you're getting an aerobic workout. These sports involve too much stopping and starting. Especially when I play, much of my time is spent picking up the balls.

STEP THREE: WEIGHT TRAINING

In weight training, knowledge is power. Unfortunately, most people don't know the most important fact: Successful weight training is the best form of exercise to reshape your body. When I weight train, I think of myself as an artist sculpting a sculpture. I spend more time on areas that need more attention, but I never forget the whole picture. If you stick to a well-rounded program created for your body, you can really change the actual shape of your physique.

The second most important fact of weight training is that it has a tremendous positive effect on your basal metabolism. Ever wonder why men seem to be able to eat much more than women and never gain an ounce? It's not the gender, it's the muscle. On the average, men have a higher muscle to fat ratio than women. It takes more calories to maintain muscle than it does to maintain fat. Therefore, if you increase the amount of muscle on your body, you increase your basal metabolism!

No one—including myself—was born with perfect symmetry, a body where all the parts match. Weight training can build the curves Mother Nature neglected to give us and create an illusion of better body proportion.

By using weight training, I was able to perfect my attributes and become a world championship bodybuilder six years in a row.

If you were born with a big rear and thunder thighs but have skinny arms, weight training can bring your butt down to size while building your arms. On the other hand, if you're top-heavy and have bird legs that only a robin would whistle at, weights can sculpt your legs into shapelier versions while toning your upper body, creating sleek symmetry. Building up one area can make another look smaller in contrast.

Bodybuilders use all sorts of tricks to sculpt their bodies to prize-winning "perfection." We put that word in quotes because like you, their bodies aren't perfect—they just look that way because they know how to play up their strengths, while downplaying the weakspots and how to stand ("pose") to hide physical flaws. Weight training is as much about creating optical illusions as muscles.

In Chapter 9, I'll share the tricks of the bodybuilding trade I relied on to win six Ms. Olympic bodybuilding championships.

Some of the greatest results of weight training are invisible: It helps fend off heart disease, high blood pressure, adult diabetes, and the brittle bones of osteoporosis.

THREE BIG FAT LIES ABOUT EXERCISE

You've heard them all so let's dismiss them for good, to eliminate confusion.

1. The Spot-Reducing Myth

All the leg lifts in the world will not burn fat directly off your legs. There's no such thing as spot reducing! The only form of exercise that actually utilizes body fat for energy is an aerobic exercise, and unfortunately it is impossible to choose where that fat is coming from. You can, however, spot shape and tone through resistance exercises so those thighs appear slimmer.

2. The Lady Godiva Myth

Worried about "getting too big" from weight training? I hear this all the time; however, women need not worry. Most of us do not have a high enough level of testosterone (male hormone) to build big, bulky muscles. If you desire a lot of muscle, it won't happen by accident. You will have to work hard, hard, hard!!!

3. The More-Is-Better Myth

Most people are under the mistaken impression that Olympic athletes exercise from the crack of dawn into the wee hours of the morning.

My coauthor was jogging seven days a week, 365 days a year, when we started to write this book. "Hey, Carole, you're running yourself into the ground," I said. "Even God rested on the seventh, so at least take one day off!"

But just as I was reluctant to turn down the volume on my bodybuilding regime for fear I'd get out of shape, she was afraid that if she stopped running every day, her muscles would quickly convert to quivering Jello.

I finally talked her into reducing her workout to five days a week. After two months, she was running faster than ever—and had lost six pounds.

She also had two extra hours a week to spend on something besides jogging—like cowriting this book, for instance. Had she kept her original pace, we might still be back on Chapter 2!

The moral of the story? More is not always better. Sometimes it's just more, sometimes it's worse.

Even though it can improve your life tremendously, getting in shape does not have to be a full-time job. As Nike elite, Michelle LeMay puts it, "There's much more to life than living in the gym. Work out to live a better life, don't live life to work out."

THE INSIDE STORY

The most miraculous thing about an exercise program is that in a matter of weeks you can have a brand new body—inside and out.

How does exercise transform a person who can barely make it around the block into someone who can knock off a six-mile run with ease—and in a matter of weeks?

As you begin exercising, your body undergoes some major changes, depending on how long, hard, fast, and often you work out—and on *how* you work out, too. As we mentioned earlier, you get what you train for. If you train for strength, you'll get stronger; if you train for speed, you'll get faster; and if you train for endurance, you'll develop enough stamina to run for miles and miles without getting winded.

Genetics is partially responsible for how you respond to training. You and a friend could follow the same training regime and progress at completely different speeds and wind up at different fitness levels—even if you're training at the same intensity. That's genetics for you; however, if you stay committed and consistent, you will both see results in as little as six weeks.

WHAT'S GOING ON INSIDE THERE?

Your heart is the biggest benefactor of exercise, which is why the American Heart Association recommends it as protection against stroke, heart disease, and even diseases triggered or aggravated by stress.

As you become more aerobically fit, your heart pumps more blood per stroke. The more blood pumped, the more oxygen that is available to your muscles. As your muscles get stronger, they are better able to extract and use the oxygen to work harder.

The left ventricle of the heart increases moderately in size because it is pumping more blood away from the heart to working muscles. At rest, your heart beats slower and has increased stroke volume.

If you also weight train, the left ventricular wall of your heart becomes thicker. Your heart must generate more force with each beat because it has to work against the increased pressure that muscle contractions put on blood vessels.

Changes usually occur within the first four to eight weeks of consistent training, and you feel your workout becoming increasingly easier.

Finally, the number of capillaries in your muscles may increase by as much as 40 percent, with more oxygen, nutrients, and hormones delivered to the muscles, and excess heat removed faster. *Aerobics* increases your muscles' ability to use oxygen for work and improves their ability to store glycogen for energy. *Weight Training* increases muscular size and strength. *Circuit Training* does both.

FAST AND SLOW TWITCHES

Muscles come in two types: fast twitch for sprintlike activities and slow twitch for endurance activities. The type of training you do determines how these muscles develop. While we're all born with a certain mix of fast and slow twitch fibers, most people have a 50-50 ratio.

Exercise does not significantly increase the number of specific fibers, but it does maximize their potential. Training for speed and power develops fast-twitch fibers while endurance training develops slow-twitch fibers.

FIFTEEN GREAT REASONS TO EXERCISE

In addition to helping you trim down, firm up, and look more symmetrical, feminine, and sexy, exercise also:

1. Builds confidence. When you're fit, you project an aura of power, strength, and self-esteem which garners respect from others and draws people to you.

2. Increases poise, balance, and coordination, especially exercises such as aerobic dance class, circuit training, and in-line skating.

3. Keeps you young. The old saying, "You're only as old as you feel," is true. Studies show that exercise makes you feel more alive and thus feel and look younger.

4. Acts as a natural tranquilizer by releasing endorphins, the "feel-good" hormone. (I love those endorphins!)

5. Helps prevent constipation, which is especially helpful for frequent flyers. When you arrive at your destination, go for a walk as soon as you check in the hotel. And drink lots of water. I swear by this routine to keep me "regular."

6. Protects against heart disease by increasing your HDL, or good cholesterol, and lowers your LDLs, or bad cholesterol.

7. Promotes strong bones and helps prevent osteoporosis.

8. Builds a stronger heart and lung capacity so you're healthier from the inside out and better able to fend off disease.

9. Reduces stress and stress-related problems, such as insomnia and anxiety. (Spoken by a person with much experience in this area!)

10. Gives your skin and hair a more youthful glow.

11. Increases your energy level. In fact, it provides an even bigger "rush" than three cups of chocolate macadamia nut gourmet cappuccino—know what I mean?

12. Increases your metabolic rate so you can eat more without gaining weight. (Confession: One reason I exercise is because I love to eat!)

13. Lowers your blood pressure and reduces your risk of stroke.

14. Increases your intellectual capacity—really! Studies show regular exercise may improve creativity, concentration, and problem solving, especially in older people.

15. Finally, exercise can open doors to new experiences and adventures you may once have lacked the strength, stamina, or confidence to enjoy. When you're in great shape, the whole world becomes your playground. You can hike to the top of the Rockies or down to the bottom of the Grand Canyon, cycle across Canada, paddle raging rivers, cross-country ski through Vermont. The sky's the limit, so why not try hang gliding? (Then again, just the thought of doing that is enough to raise my pulse. Maybe I'll pass on that one!)

EXERCISE AND KIDS

We know that exercise is great for adults. But what about for kids? Studies show that 40 percent of children ages five to eight exhibit at least one high-risk factor of heart disease.

While no specific guidelines for kids have been established because little research has been done, experts recommend a half hour of noncompetitive, "fun" exercise every day to reduce the risks of childhood obesity, high blood pressure, and high cholesterol. Also, because atherosclerosis starts in childhood, regular exercise helps prevent the onset of this and other degenerative diseases.

As far as weight training, experts agree that children should wait to do full weight training until their bodies are fully matured and their bones have completed the growth period and ossification process.

Children should never perform weight-bearing exercises like heavy squats or overhead lifts, which puts compression forces on the spine.

Also, because kids' bodies are not as efficient at regulating internal heat, they should not exercise for a long time at high intensity. Injuries and repeated stress can stunt a child's growth by damaging the bone cartilage that monitors height, as children's bones are not completely fused until sometime in late adolescence.

If you have children and are concerned about safe exercising, why not enroll together in a Mommy-and-me program and get fit together? Or develop your own fitness program and you'll get to know your kids in a brand-new way. Or look into exercise videos just for kids. Whatever you do, make it fun, and your kids will be exercising without whining. In fact, they'll beg you to let them "play."

A STRETCH IN TIME

As we mentioned above, all workouts should begin with a warm-up and end with a cool-down. My choreographer, Michelle LeMay, who helped develop the Nike stretch program, recommends light stretching in the warm-up and deeper stretching in the cool-down. She says the purpose of stretching in the warm-up is to loosen your muscles, lubricate your joints, and prepare you for the workout that follows. The cool-down is where you can really enhance flexibility. Your muscles are nice and warm from your workout and therefore more pliable and ready for a deeper stretch.

RANGE OF MOTION

One phrase you'll hear a lot concerning stretching is range of motion, which refers to how far your body naturally moves in a given direction. Touching your toes is a normal range of motion whereas swiveling your head around Exorcist-style is definitely not—unless you happen to be Linda Blair.

The aim of all stretching programs is to gradually increase your range of motion so you're more flexible and limber. Even if you can't touch your knees today, after a few months of stretching you'll be able to touch your toes or even lay your hands flat on the ground.

NINE TIPS FOR SAFE STRETCHING

1. Never force a move. It takes time to develop flexibility, and pushing your body to go in a direction it's not limber enough to achieve could result in soreness or injury.

2. Never stretch a cold muscle. Warm muscles are more pliable and safer to stretch.

3. Stretch every muscle group before exercising: calves, hamstrings, quadriceps, hip flexors, rotators, lower back extensors, chest, and shoulder muscles.

4. Never hold your breath when stretching; your body requires an even exchange of oxygen, and holding your breath tends to make you tense up. Just breathe naturally, relax, and go with the flow.

5. Don't bounce. Save the "ballistics" for the movies. Stretch slow and in complete control without momentum or body weight dictating the degree of the stretch.

Stretch to the point of mild discomfort in the belly of the muscle. If you feel discomfort at or near the joint area, increase the bend at the joint and ease up if necessary.

6. As your flexibility increases, move farther into your natural range of motion, continuing to stretch smoothly and evenly without bouncing.

7. Don't ever attempt dangerous stretches or the sort of weird contortions you see at the circus. Those guys are trained acrobatics—and many of them are double-jointed besides. Just because Jean Claude Van Damme can wrap his leg behind his head 10 times doesn't mean you or I can.

8. The following stretches are dangerous. Never do them:

- full-squat bouncing stretches
- hurdle stretches.
- lower-back stretches with your knees locked
- stretching your back by rolling up and back on your neck (the Plow).

9. Wake up and stretch—whether you're planning to exercise that day or not. You'll feel more alive, and a daily stretch will protect you from injuring yourself during everyday "bad moves" such as lifting too many files at work, or suddenly twisting when you're holding a squirming infant, or common mistakes like picking up luggage with straight legs.

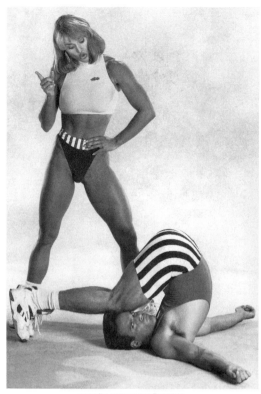

UNSAFE EXERCISE
Stretch no-nos: never stretch by rolling up on your neck.

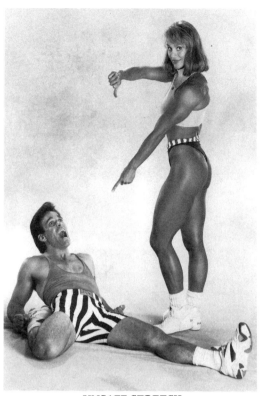

UNSAFE STRETCH
Hurdler stretches put too much pressure on the knees. Don't do it.

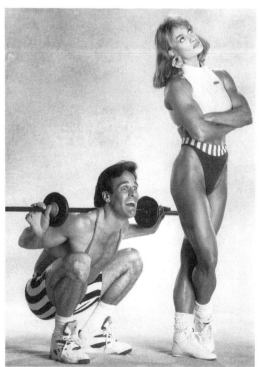

IMPROPER TECHNIQUE
"Okay, Mr. Smart Guy. How many times have I told you not to squat with your thighs below your knees. This is murder on the knees."

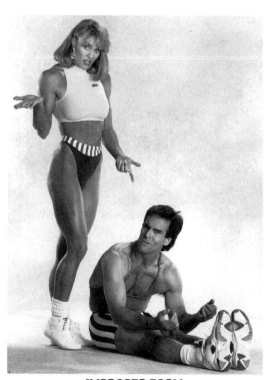

IMPROPER FORM
Don't lock your knees when you do a lower back and hamstring stretch. Keep your knees slightly bent so you feel it in the belly of the muscle.

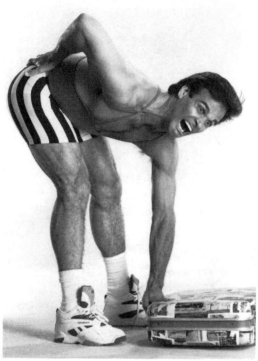

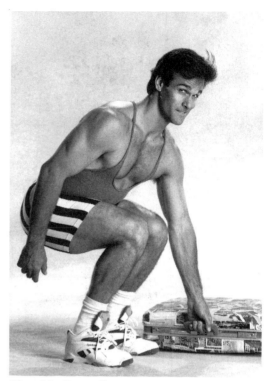

Talk about a bad move. Mr. Smart Guy here is going to wind up with a very sore back.

Okay, Mr. Smart Guy—you did it right!

Here's a great stretching workout for you do do at home.

Cory's Daily Stretch

It's more fun to stretch with a partner—always follow proper form as discussed earlier, never bounce or jerk. A partner can give you additional resistance in all your stretches to increase your flexibility and range of motion. Have your partner hold you in a comfortable stretching position for 10 seconds, then slowly release all pressure. Repeat with slow, slight pressure for 10 seconds, and repeat again.

1. Hamstrings, low back, and calf.
2. Quadriceps and Hip flexor
3. Hip flexor
4. Calf stretch
5. Ankles
6. Hip rotator (Deep lateral rotators)
7. Adductors (Butterfly stretch), (Straddle stretch)
8. Forearm
9. Chest (seated), (standing)
10. Shoulder
11. Neck
12. Arms (seated), (standing)

In the following chapters, we'll give you the lowdown on aerobics, plus eight different workouts to keep you from getting bored or stuck in an exercise rut. Mix 'em, match 'em, or pick your favorite and go for it. It's your choice, and with 64 different workouts you'll have plenty of options. In Chapter 9, I'll tell you everything you always wanted to know about how to weight train your way to a stronger and more shapely body. Good luck—and stay motivated!

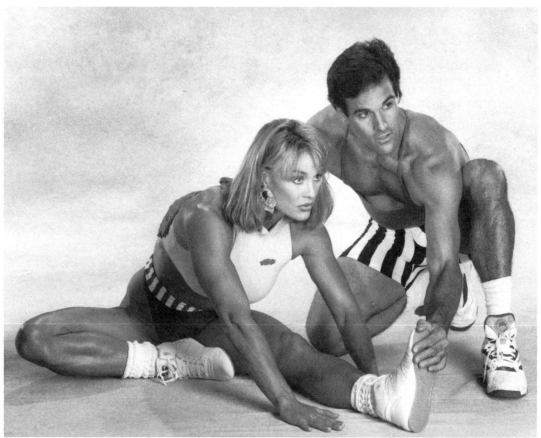

Inverted hurdler stretch: Good stretch for hamstring and lower back and calf muscles. Keep your back straight, bring your stomach to your thigh keeping your knee slightly bent so you feel it in the belly of the hamstring and not in the knee joint.

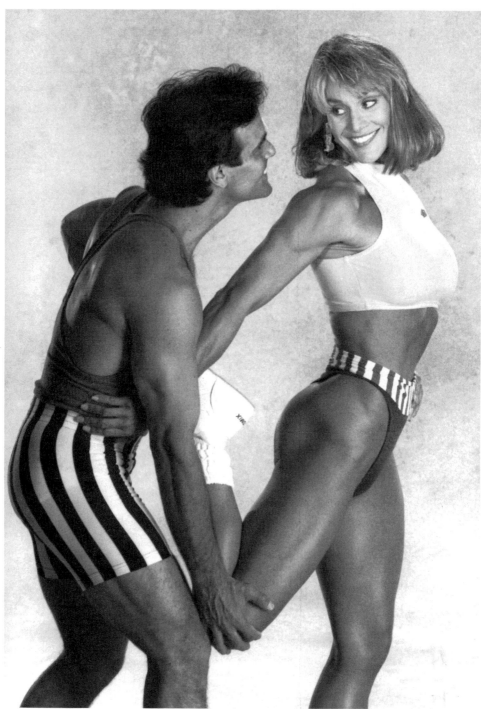

A good quadricep and hip flexor stretch, but know your limitations. Communication is important when you stretch with a partner. (All stretches can be done on your own.)

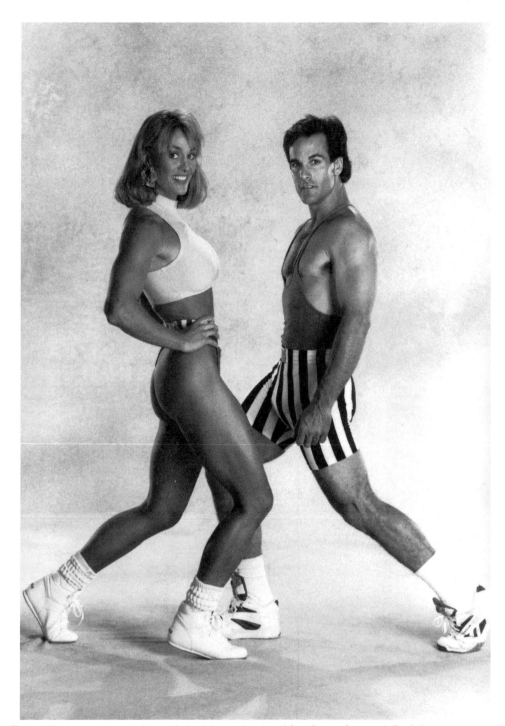

Hip flexor: Tuck your hips under with both knees bent and feet facing forward. Feel the stretch in the hip flexor of the back leg.

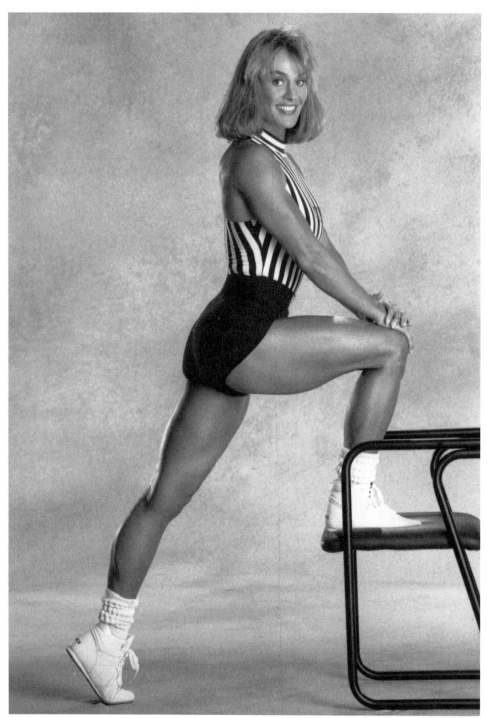

Calf stretch: Be sure your toes are facing forward and gently press your heel to the floor.

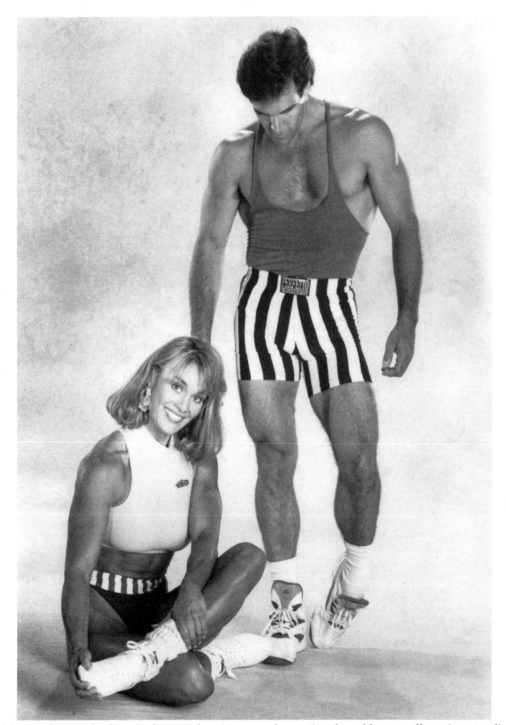

Ankle stretches can be done in the seated position, gently rotating the ankle manually, or in a standing position, rotating the ankle on the floor.

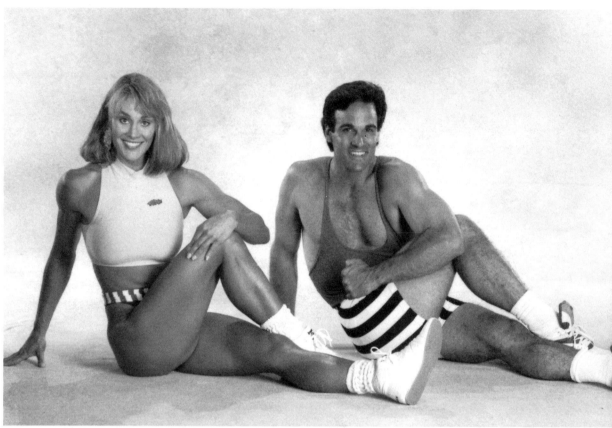

This position stretches your hips. Gently pull your knee to your chest for an increased stretch.

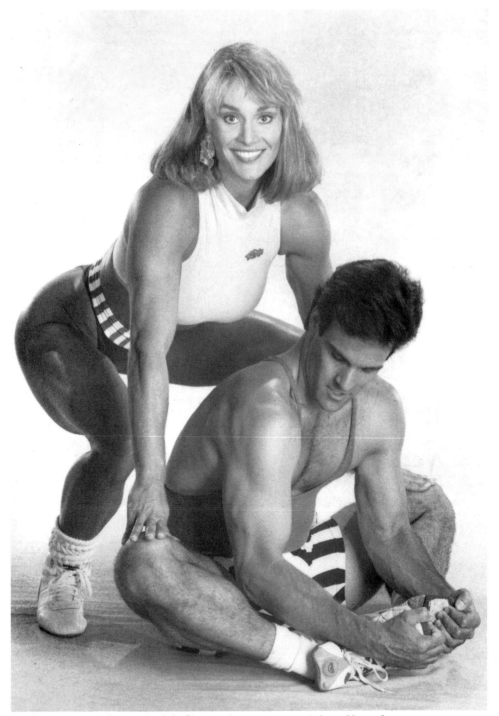

Seated adductor stretch (inner thighs): Slow and easy pressure is best. Never force your partner to go further than what is comfortable.

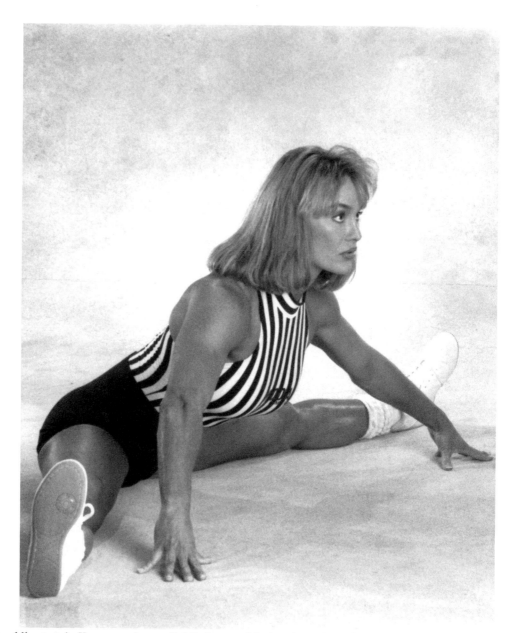

Straddle stretch: Keep your knees slightly bent and facing the ceiling. Go only to the point of mild discomfort.

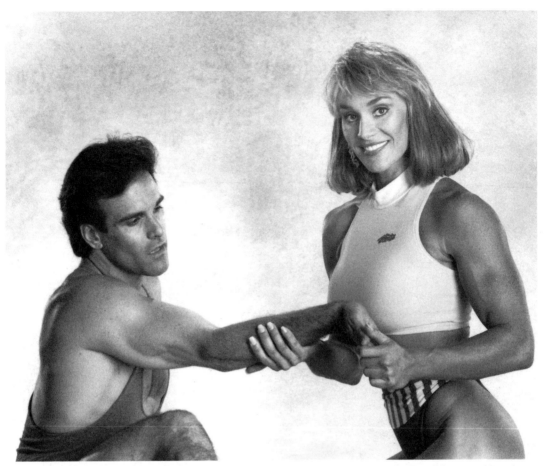

Forearm stretch: Especially good for racquet sports and occupations that require lots of arm and hand use.

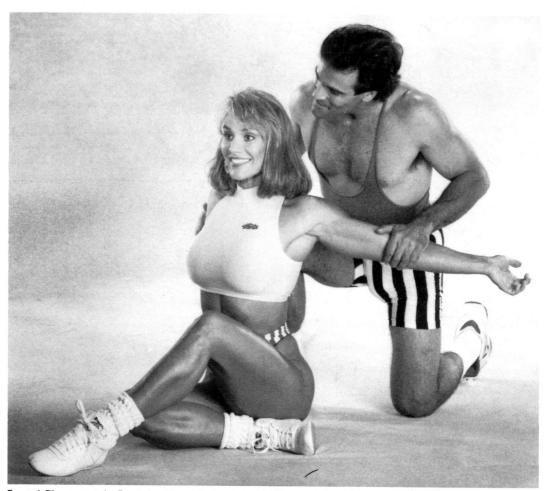

Seated Chest stretch: Stretches the anterior deltoids (front of shoulders) along with the pectorals.

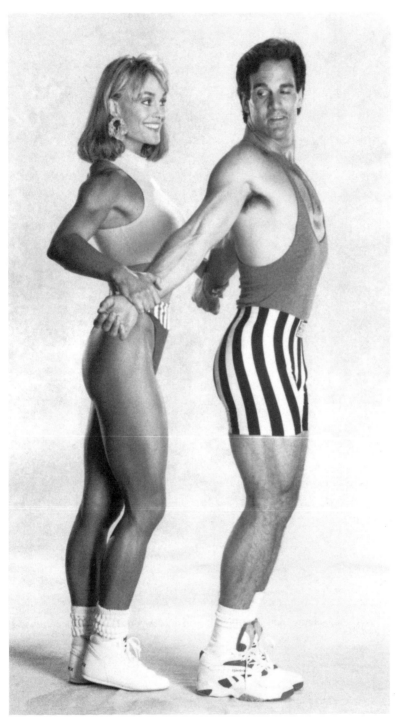

Standing chest stretch: Stretches the anterior deltoid along with the pectorals. This illustrates a different angle from the previous stretch. I recommend stretching through both angles for increased range of motion.

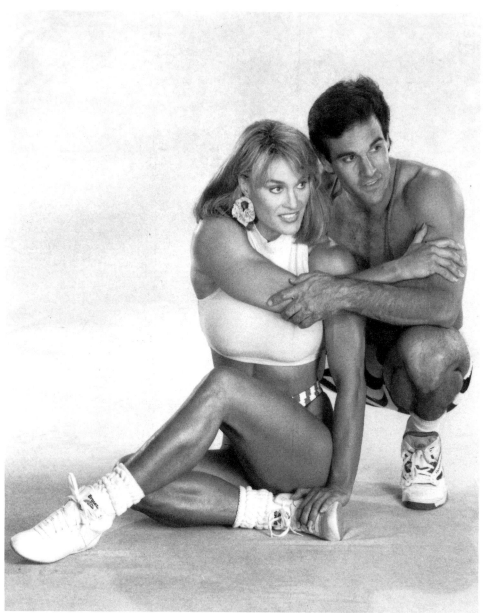

Shoulder stretch: Have your partner gently pull your arm across your body at the elbow to stretch the rear deltoid.

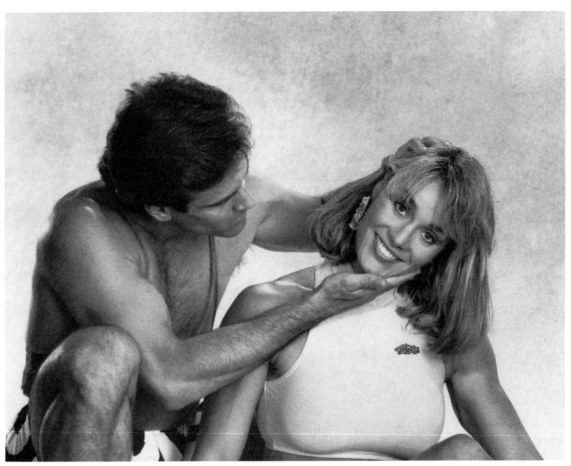

"Be careful, Mr. Smart Guy. My neck is fragile."

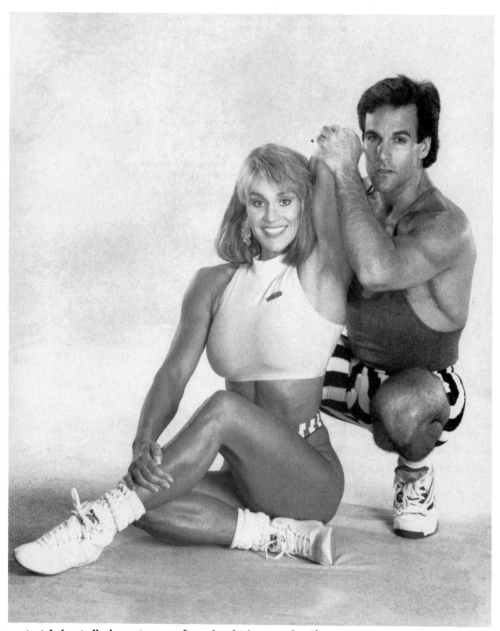

Tricep stretch (seated): A great move after a hard tricep workout!

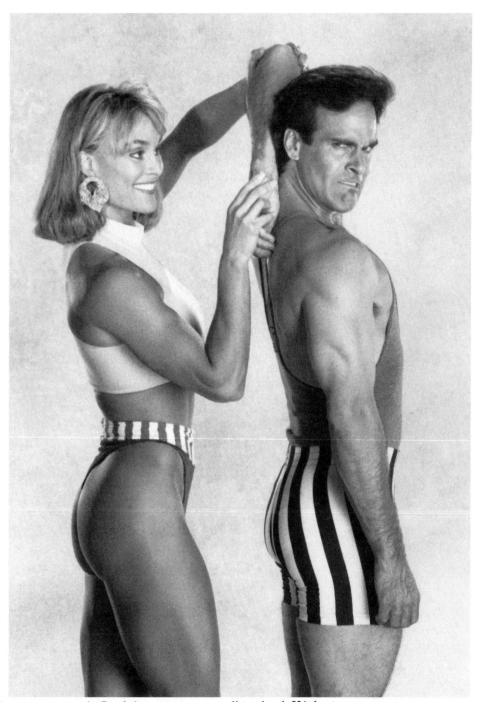

Standing triceps stretch. Don't let your partner pull too hard. If it hurts, ease up.

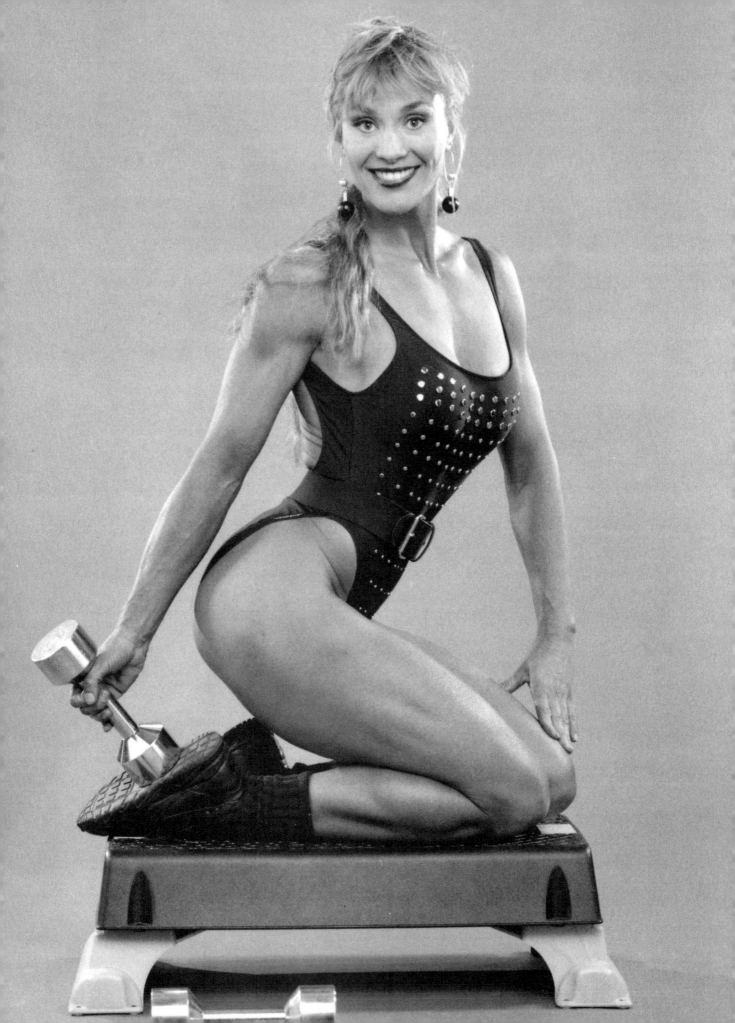

Seven

Everything You Ever Wanted to Know About Aerobics

Exercise is flab's worst enemy—and a girl's best friend. But here's a deep, dark secret most exercise buffs rarely 'fess up to: Many of them absolutely hated exercise when they first started. Maybe just like you, they grumped and groaned their way to their workouts and came up with every excuse on earth to wriggle out of it. But within a matter of weeks they were hooked.

Why? In a word, RESULTS.

So here's the skinny on getting started, ladies: You don't have to adore exercise to begin; in fact, feel free to hate it at first. Within a matter of weeks you'll be eyeing the clock for the minute you can skip off to the gym—or maybe even setting your alarm at 6 A.M. to rise and shine with aerobics. Even better, you'll be smiling instead of scowling in the mirror.

Fat chance, you say? Well, give this program a month and you won't believe your eyes. Not only will you have muscles where you once had lumps, but new curves where you never thought to look for them. All the while, you'll be turning fat into an out-of-body experience. And talk about stamina, you'll be raring to go, whether it's to the gym or off to work.

When that light bulb flashes in your mind and you realize that exercise isn't something you can take or leave, but an essential part of your life—like breathing, or going to work every day (or for me, painting)—you'll have it made.

Not only will you no longer dread exercise, you'll actually look forward to it as the miracle it is and wonder how you ever managed without it.

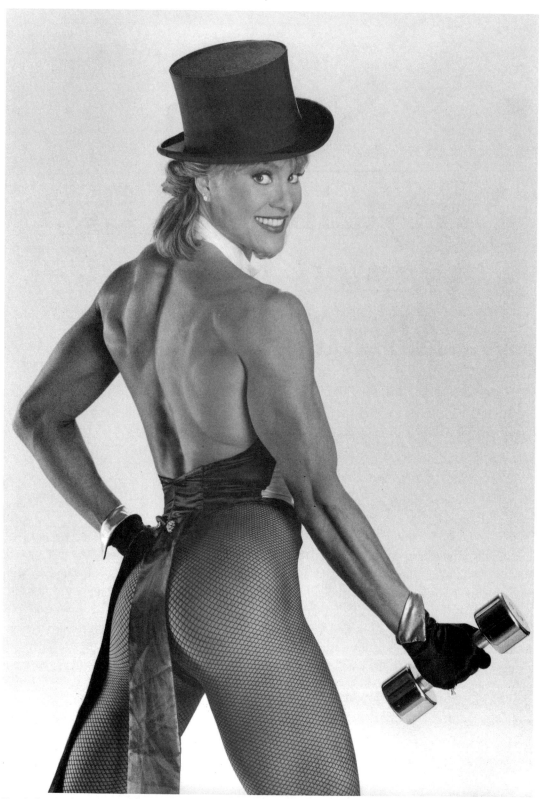

Don't let the holidays slow you down and fatten you up. Your workout will help you enjoy the holidays more than ever.

IT DON'T MEAN A THING IF IT AIN'T GOT THAT ZING

So which is the best exercise? People are always surprised at my reply: "The one you like best!" It's not the one that burns the most calories or works up the biggest sweat, but the one you enjoy so much you can't wait to lace up and go-go-go.

Take my co-author, for example. She loves in-line skating so much that her boss has threatened to wire her with a pager. Once she rolls out that door at noon, there's no telling when she'll roll back. Hours pass; one day she didn't return until her comrades had left for the day.

"It's true," Carole chuckles. "Once I buckle up my Lightning skates—Whee—I'm free again and reliving my childhood. I can hardly bare to take them off."

Exercise? Well sure it's that, too, but Carole swears that's besides the point. While in-line skating burns tons of calories and has given her buns of steel and killer thighs, Carole assures me, "The main reason I do it is because it's a total blast and the high point of my day."

Find an exercise program you love that much, and you'll be on a fitness roll. Not that you have to settle on just one. The more the merrier! Be a little fickle and you'll enjoy a host of fitness benefits. Mix and match to your heart's content. You'll not only have more fun but also be far less injury-prone because you won't be using the same muscles all the time. Besides, cross-training will keep you motivated. Variety is the spice of life, remember? Eat the same thing for dinner every night? Hardly. Your exercise life should be no exception. The same ole' same ole' day after day sets the stage for exercise burnout and dropout.

UPPING THE ANTE

One day, you wake up as usual, do your workout, and nothing happens. No burn, no sweat— the truth is you could have done it in your sleep.

It's hard to believe, but that killer workout you once sweated and groaned through has lost its aerobic feeling. In fact, it's become downright . . . (could it be true?) . . . easy!

This fact of exercise life is called the training plateau. Even if you don't think it could happen to you in a million years, trust me—it can and will happen to any woman who sticks to the program.

There's only one way to climb out of a plateau, and that's to shake up your workout. You do this by adjusting intensity or duration—or both. Note that we didn't say add but adjust.

A friend of mine panicked when faced with her first plateau. "Okay, I'll do more, but do I have to keep doing more and more and more and . . . ?"

According to Phillip Walker at the Cooper Clinic, the idea is to adjust your workout by baby steps, not leaps and bounds. Add a few yards here, shave a few seconds there, until you reach a level that feels like your peak.

We're *not* saying you have to keep upping the ante until you qualify for the Olympics, rather just until you reach a level that's comfortable for you, and lets you accomplish your fitness dream—whether it's running a three-mile fun run or the Boston marathon.

When you reach your dream peak, you have two choices: You can maintain your current workout and stay there, or take a week or two off, start back in the middle, and work up again, repeating the process for the rest of your life.

THE PROBLEM WITH THE STATUS QUO

Settle into that plateau and not only will you not get more fit, but you may get fatter.

Walker often counsels women who are understandably upset. They think he won't believe them when they say they're gaining weight while running five miles a day and eating what they should.

Walker believes them all right. In fact he sees it all the time—and it's the "running five miles for years now" that raises his red flag. "Same route?" he asks. "Yep!" they reply. "Same number of miles per day?" "Yep!" "Same pace throughout?" "Yep!"

Mystery solved, he says. Your body becomes so used to your workout that the minute you lace up your Nikes it begins yawning. "Here we go again," it says, punching the snooze button on your metabolism. "Wake me up when it's over."

No wonder you're gaining weight, he tells them. Your body has grown so accustomed to the same old workout that it can do it in its sleep.

MORE IS NOT, WE REPEAT, BETTER

Rather than asking them to run more, which is what they all fear, Walker simply adjusts their workouts to alternate between "push" and "cruise" cycles, or what's called interval training or "fartlek." (No connection to . . . well, you know.)

In a month or so these women not only lose weight but are running better than ever before the same or fewer miles they had been gaining weight on before. A miracle? Nope—they have simply awakened a slumbering metabolism.

Walker uses the same principle on himself with great success. Before he took his current job at the Cooper Clinic where he basically sits for eight hours, Walker trained eight hours a day as an Olympic cross-country skier. To avoid gaining weight after leaving competition, he developed a condensed, power-packed workout that mimicked his eight-hour training day, but over a week: Twice a week, Walker runs two miles hard and fast; another two days he jogs five to six miles at comfortable pace. And on the fifth day, he jogs 20 miles. The result? Walker hasn't gained an ounce in years although he exercises only a fraction of what he did as an Olympian.

Just for fun, a few months from now, drop back to the routine you're starting with now. Whether it's running two miles or pressing 10 pounds, you won't believe how easy it is compared to how hard it once seemed. Honest!

SLOWER IS FASTER

Remember the tortoise and the hare? This is no fairytale, ladies. It also applies to your exercise program.

Experts agree that exercising for a longer period of time at a slower pace, as in speedwalking or slow jogging, burns more fat than blasts of exercise like sprinting. Since most of us can walk much farther than we can jog, and jog a lot farther than we can run, going slower is often far better than speeding.

Whether you run that mile or walk it, you'll burn about the same number of calories.

BURNING FAT BY STAYING ON TARGET

To turn on your fat-burning furnace while you are exercising, you must do an an activity considered to be "aerobic." An aerobic exercise is one in which you work out consistently for 20–60 minutes in your THR (Target Heart Rate) range. It is recommended that you do this at least three times a week.

Your target heart rate range gives you a training zone of safe, effective exercise pulse rates, based on your age and level of fitness. To achieve an aerobic effect, you must keep your heart rate between 60 and 90 percent of its maximum. To find your target heart rate range, you'll want to calculate both 60 and 90 percent of your maximum heart rate to find the low and high ends of your range. Your pulse rate will vary, but try to stay within this range to maintain an aerobic effect.

Below is a general formula to find a safe THR range; however, while this formula does incorporate your age, it does not incorporate your fitness level. Mark Santella, exercise physiologist for fitness systems, explains: "Target heart rate is population-specific. There are many important factors to consider such as age, weight, fitness level, and individual fitness goals. An athlete who desires a maximum aerobic gain will train in a different area of their THR range than someone who simply wants to maintain her health and burn a little body fat."

Start with the formula below and as you get more serious about your exercise program, you may want to get more specific in your training zone. At that point, see your local certified trainer or certified aerobics instructor to help you hone in on the specifics. A good rule of thumb to follow—if you are a beginner, begin exercising at the lower end of your THR range. As you progress and begin to hit plateaus, you can increase your intensity so that you will continue to get results. Just remember, if you're looking for aerobic benefits, exercising under or over your THR range won't allow you to reap those fabulous benefits of aerobic-exercise.

Here's how to find your training range:

1. Start with 220. Subtract your age. Let's say you're 30. The result, 190, is your predicted maximum safe heart rate. Forty years old? Your maximum is 180. Now try it: 220 − ___ = ___.
2. For the low end of your range, multiply your maximum rate by .60 for 60 percent (low end equals 114 for age 30). For you: ___ × .6 = ___.
3. For the high end of your range, multiply by .9 for 90 percent (high end equals 171 for age 30). So: ___ × .9 = ___.
4. Divide by six to find your 10-second heart rate for high or low rates. (114 divided by 6 equals 19). Your high rate: ___ / 6 = ___. Your low rate: ___ / 6 = ___.

Beginners should work at the low end and only competing athletes should aim for the high end.

To take your pulse:

1. Use your first two fingers, not your thumb. Press lightly on your radial artery, close to your other thumb on the inside of your wrist, or on the carotid artery of your neck, straight down from the corner of your eye and just under your chin.
2. Count the number of beats for 10 seconds and multiply by 6.
3. Check your pulse rate periodically throughout your workout and right after finishing the aerobic portion. If your pulse is within range, maintain the intensity. If it's too high, slow your pace. Too low? Speed up.

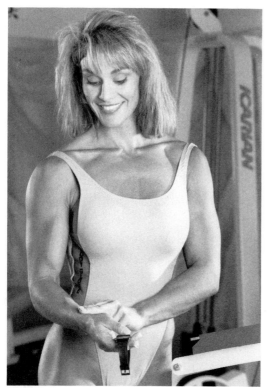

Find your pulse in your radial artery on the inside of your wrist.

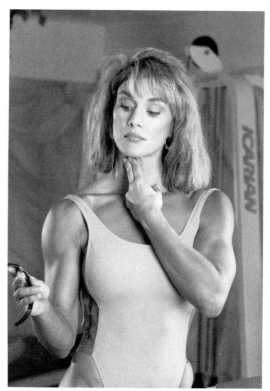

Find your pulse in your carotid artery in your neck.

Remember, exercise is supposed to make you feel healthier, not worse. In time, you'll know what your "right" target feels like, and you won't have to bother taking your pulse. But for beginners, this method is an accurate way to maintain a pace that's not only safe but which also builds aerobic capacity—and burns fat.

You know you're overdoing it if your chest starts pounding like crazy or if you feel dizzy or faint. Just cool down for about 5 to 10 minutes before ending your workout. If this keeps up, and you're working below your high rate, see a doctor.

ELECTRONIC COACHES

If this math is too much for you, buy a heart-rate monitor. These handy little gadgets provide an instant readout of your heart rate as you exercise. Some are waterproof for swimmers. It's like having a coach in your back pocket.

The most accurate monitors are chest monitors; these read the pulse via sensors attached to a chest strap transmitted to a watchlike device. Some are specifically made for cycling and mount on handlebars.

Prices range from about $120 to $450; some "beep" when you're exercising too hard or too little. Others transfer your vital signs during exercise to a personal computer to provide a permanent record.

More affordable than chest monitors but less accurate are models whose sensors attach to your earlobes or fingertips, while the receiver clips to your shirt. Average price is about $50.

As well as eliminating the math, by offering a continuous readout while you're exercising, monitors let you compare the benefits of various workouts so you can nail down the most burn for your effort.

AEROBICS TO GO-GO

Now that you know how to exercise safely within your training zone, let's look at a few of my favorite ways to move it!

Speedwalking (about 4½ miles per hour)

My number-one aerobics choice, speedwalking is ideal for novices. Just lace up and walk quickly, swinging your arms. While the waddlelike walk may look more like Donald Duck at times, this exercise is no quack. It's easy, safe, and something you can do anywhere, anytime (unless there's snow on the ground).

It's also perfect for those who can't afford gyms or wouldn't be caught dead in one, although some of us fare better with a walking buddy. Mine is Bolaro, my giant schnauser, who keeps my pulse up there.

Teaming up not only keeps you from dropping out, but will give you a motivational soulmate who can share your accomplishments. For those of you who prefer solitude, speedwalking lets you walk away from it all (your job, boss, boyfriend, the kids) and return in 30 minutes feeling like a new woman. Walk to your favorite music—the faster the beat, the faster you walk.

Because speedwalking uses the round, rhythmic motions of large muscle groups, you'll hit a steady cadence that soothes the body, quiets your nerves, and helps you concentrate. Situations that seemed impossibly tangled become crystal clear, and your creativity soars. I can't tell you how many ideas for books, videos, art, scripts, even home improvement plans, I've brainstormed while walking. Ask Bolaro! I talk it all over with him.

PMS got you down? Take a hike or walk. Nothing on earth eases depression faster than a brisk walk.

Aerobic Dance

Here's a musical way to shake, rattle, and roll off fat. Whether it's funk aerobics, jazz, or rocking to the oldies, aerobic dance strengthens muscles, develops balance and coordination, and it's just plain fun. Start a library of dance videos and turn your living room into your personal dance studio.

Step Aerobics

This is my favorite type of aerobic dance. You step up and down on a block—as if you were climbing an endless set of bleachers using dancelike moves and music.

Step shapes hips, thighs, stomach, and buns while increasing your cardiovascular capacity.

Years ago, before step became popular, we did our own homegrown version on wooden benches on the playing fields. If I had known then how popular step would become one day, I would have invented a step back then and become an overnight millionaire.

Most health clubs offer step workouts, or you can purchase a step and a few videos and do it at home.

I've produced three step videos that will have you stepping high in no time flat: *Cory Everson's Step 'N Time, Total Body Workout,* and *Step Training,* as well as a step called Cory's Step Trainer. For more information, call (708) 855-0294 and ask about the package price. Or see the video listings at the end of this chapter.

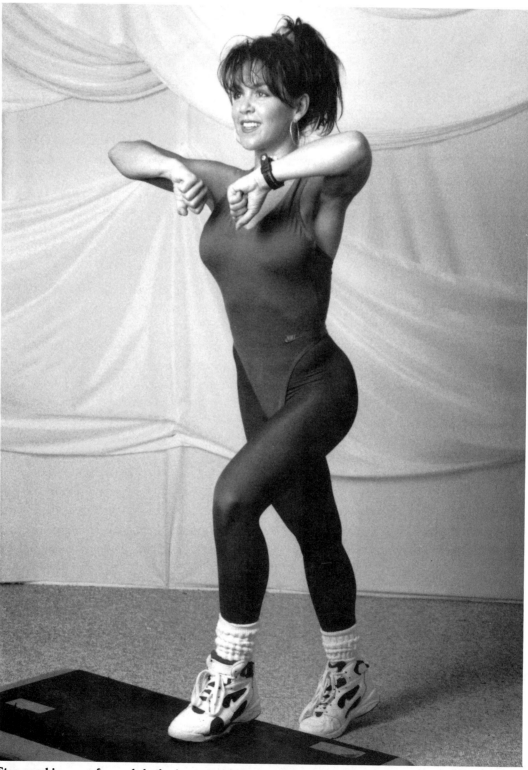

Step aerobics are a fun and rhythmic way to shake your bootie—and firm the bod—as demonstrated by Michelle LeMay.

Jogging (about 5½ miles per hour)

You've no doubt heard the controversy over jogging with many people claiming it ruined their knees and made their breasts sag. The fact is, running can be highly injurious to joints and knees if you wear the wrong shoes or take on too much distance too soon. Despite these drawbacks, hundreds of thousands of people manage to jog safely and effectively and running has become an important part of their lives. And with good reason: Running is an excellent fat burner and a terrific way to boost cardiovascular strength—not to mention the "runner's high" some people feel after a few months into their training.

My advice is to approach running enthusiastically, but with caution—take it slow at first and see if it's right for you. If you have a prior foot or leg injury, running may very well aggravate it. If you have any bio-mechanical imbalance, running will find it. If this is the case, you should perhaps opt for a lower impact (or no impact) activity such as cycling or swimming.

Before you take one step, invest in a pair of quality running shoes which will go a long way toward cushioning the impact. Good shoes will cost at least $60, but believe me, the money will be well spent. Those old Keds just won't make it!

A good jogging bra is another worthwhile investment, and something you can wear for hiking, cycling, etc. While studies show that jogging doesn't contribute to sagging breasts, the bouncing may irritate you, and a jogging bra will give you some needed support.

Start slow, perhaps combining jogging with walking at first. Don't push too hard; do what feels comfortable at first and allow your muscles to adjust to this new activity. Expect some soreness initially and remember to stretch thoroughly both before and after.

If you experience sharp pain to any joints, stop. The old adage, "no pain, no gain," does not apply here. Pain means something is wrong, and if you continue to run with pain, you will most likely bring on injury.

If possible, run at least once a week or more on soft surfaces and avoid running downhill on hard pavement. Start with a half mile and add no more than 10 percent more distance per week. Even if you feel like you can do more, take it slowly. Most new runners suffer an injury after a couple of months, just when they're starting to feel strong and they overdo it. Unless you're training for a marathon, keep your weekly mileage to under 20 to 25 miles to minimize injuries.

Swimming

Because swimming uses all your muscles, it provides more of an overall conditioning effect than jogging or speedwalking. It's also the perfect workout if you've been injured, since the buoyancy of the water trims pressure on your bones and joints. On the downside, you must belong to a health club with a pool, which may not be convenient. Some complain that chlorine irritates eyes (good goggles can prevent this) and dries out skin and hair. If you intend to use swimming as your primary aerobic exercise, swim in heated pools. Swimming in cold water may slow your metabolism, telling your body to hold onto or even create fat reserves to insulate you from the cold water. (No wonder whales have so much blubber.) Also, many women find that swimming is a bit too relaxing in mid-day. My co-author tried it for a while, and by 3 P.M. she was nodding off at her computer. Personally, I once swam a lot—and it never helped me lose weight. But to each her own. While not as aerobic as jogging, swimming surpasses speedwalking and aerobics for calorie burn, and you can swim up to 10 miles a day without doing any damage to your joints. On the other hand, you have to be a technically good swimmer to work up a "sweat." Otherwise, you'll wind up fighting the water and tire before you can burn many calories.

Cycling

Because cycling puts less strain on joints and muscles, it's perfect for those who can't jog because of prior injuries. To get an aerobic effect, pedal steadily at 15 miles per hour. Don't just cruise along. Downhill rides offer a nice breather and time to enjoy the view, but zilch aerobic benefits. You can also cover a lot of ground on a bicycle, enabling you to vary your course and keep it interesting.

Mountain Biking

Off-road cycling offers an even better workout than regular cycling because the bicycle weighs more and its fatter tires offer more resistance. The nature of the ride forces you to use your entire body to steer, offering more of a total-body workout. Because mountain bikes were built to go where skinny tires fear to tread—through streams, gullies, and sand—they offer a grueling workout that uses every muscle in your body. You can even use your mountain bike in the snow as long as you bundle up carefully.

In-line Skating (10 miles per hour)

Who says you can't reinvent the wheel? Remember those rollerskates from yesteryear? Today's new skates provide a much smoother ride and a workout that's vigorous and fun.

While not quite as aerobic as running, especially if you roll along rather than skate hard, and not as efficient for toning and shaping muscles as weight training, in-line skating is a great overall workout, with an aerobic burn somewhere between cycling and running. If you make in-line skating your primary aerobic sport, skate vigorously for 75 to 90 minutes three times a week. But be careful. This sport can be dangerous if you tackle hills before you master stopping. We highly recommend lessons, knee and elbow pads, wrist guards, and helmets. I should have a butt guard, as my stopping technique involves landing on my derriere.

Once you learn in-line skating and figure out how to stop without falling, it may become dangerously addictive—so much fun you can't stop. The breeze cools the sweat so you hardly notice you're working out. For a maximum workout, stride for 15 minutes, push hard for a minute, and repeat the sequence. A 75-minute skate qualifies as one training day. Nothing on earth is better for toning and firming your butt, inner thigh, and low back muscles.

Cross-country Skiing

Cross-country skiing uses every major muscle, and, because the weather is cold, your body burns more calories just keeping you warm.

Cross-country is the best workout you can get on land or water. Particularly aerobic is cross-country skating, which looks like ice skating on skis.

Boxing

You know. Like, right hook, boom! Left hook, boom! If you thought boxing was just for the guys, put up your dukes. Adopt a boxing-based fitness program and your fat won't have a fighting chance. Health clubs across the country now offer boxing-aerobics. You get all the fitness

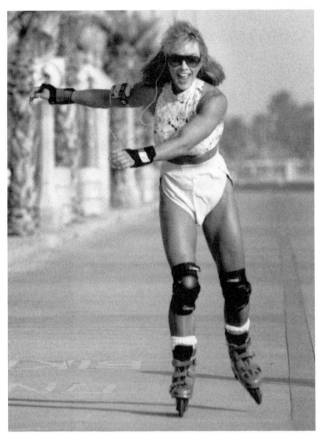

Who says you can't reinvent the wheel? In-line
skating puts you on a real aerobic roll.

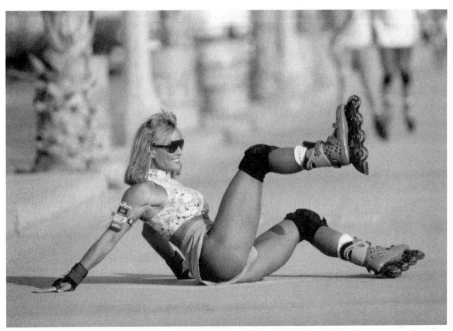

Unfortunately, this is where I usually wind up. Play it safe by taking lessons, and wear wrist guards, knee
pads, and a helmet to protect yourself from injuries.

benefits of boxing minus the black eye—since the only one you ever "punch out" is yourself, in the mirror, that is. ("I shouldn't have eaten that Snickers! Boom!")

Although programs vary, a typical workout begins with 10 minutes of stretching, followed by several rounds of jumping rope, then 10 to 20 minutes of punching drills where you hit a big, sausagelike bag to increase body strength. If it helps motivate you, think of your ex, your boss, or your mother-in-law. Just kidding, Mom!

Sliding

Also called lateral motion training, sliding is a workout staple for speed skaters, skiers, and hockey players who train indoors on "slide boards," those slick plastic mats 6 to 8 feet across and about 2 feet wide that are creeping into health clubs and home gyms.

Although it takes practice, sliding involves wearing slippery nylon boots over sneakers, then pushing off against the mat's end blocks, sliding from side to side in the same motion used in speed skating. The repeated leg flexing raises your pulse while giving your inner and outer thighs, buttocks, and knee muscles a great workout. Professional hockey, skiing, and racquetball teams have also taken to sliding to improve performance.

All but the biggest boards roll up into light, tight tubes with carrying straps. Reebok is introducing a Slide Reebok nationally, so stay tuned for slide classes at your local gym.

Kneedspeed also sells quality boards aimed at aerobic exercisers and includes a 30-minute workout. Call (800) 523-7674 for information.

A WORD ON CROSS-TRAINING

It's just what it sounds like—mixing and matching everything from hiking to cycling so you don't get bored. It's most efficient when you combine activities that fill each other's gaps. For in-

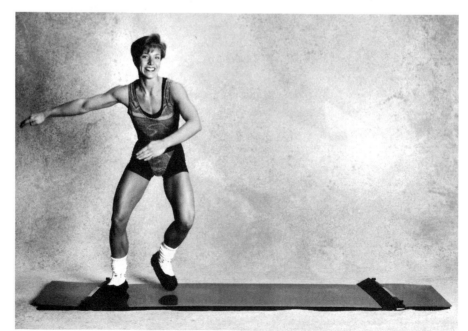

No buts about it: Sliding, a trendy new workout used by speed skaters and other athletes, really works your butt.

stance, combine two aerobic activities like jogging and rowing for a total lower (jogging) and upper (rowing) body workout.

While keeping you balanced in a physical sense, cross-training keeps you on an even emotional and mental keel by taking off the pressure and offering you lots of aerobic choices. Too pooped to run? No problem. Take a leisurely spin on your bike or a nice, long walk. This is exactly what I do, especially when I'm on the road or too busy for an official workout at the gym. Consider each day a game and ask yourself, "How do I feel like playing today?"

LEAN, MEAN MACHINES

We'd need an encyclopedia to rate all the exercise equipment out there, so we've limited our discussion to our top choices. To ensure you work all your major muscle groups, do as I do and machine hop. It's fun, it keeps things interesting and wow! What a workout!

Stair Climbers

Probably the best calorie-burner of the machine bunch, and with all the new computerized programs you can climb mountains all over the world without leaving the gym. Stand straight up (leaning forward could tighten muscles in your legs and strain your knees or back). Rest your arms on the side rails—don't lock your elbows to support yourself. Finally, make sure the footpads aren't worn out. Place your feet hip-width apart so they don't swing too much and use short strides.

Treadmills

A great way to take a nice, long walk or jog rain or shine. While treadmills don't offer the same aerobic benefits as jogging because there's less resistance, you can vary the speed to increase the caloric burn.

Just don't go too fast, and make sure the machine has an emergency stop switch and a side railing. For safety's sake, before you start to walk straddle the tread so you don't get jolted (or thrown) to a quick start. Turn on the machine to a slow pace and step onto the tread, holding the railings. Once you're balanced, move off with a brisk walk, arms swinging comfortably at your sides. Gradually progress to a faster walk or jog, striding just as you would outdoors.

By adding arm motion, you'll increase the caloric burn. When you're ready to quit, gradually turn down the speed of the sidewalk until you're walking very slowly, and wait for a complete stop before stepping off.

Stationary Bicycles

You may not have the scenic stimulation of outdoor riding, but you do have resistance control right at your fingertips. Unless you have a straight stretch without stop signs, crosswalks, and hills, outdoor biking can be filled with various interruptions to your aerobic workout.

Adjust the seat so you have a slight bend in your knee at the bottom pedal position, and so you're neither reaching for the pedal nor bringing your knees up too high. Then adjust the handlebars so they're comfortable. Drive the pedals with each of your legs rather than applying force with your upper body or swinging your hips from side to side as you stroke. Keep your upper body relatively still. Make a circle with your pedaling, pushing with the ball of each foot. Otherwise you'll wind up with a real pain in the butt.

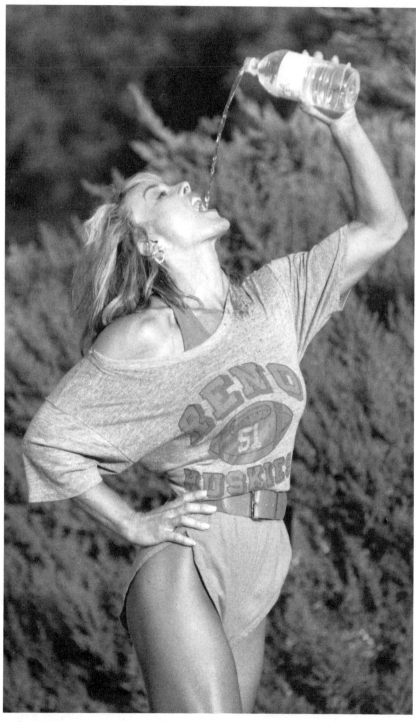

Drink plenty of water before working out. The best replenisher for most workouts is still H$_2$O.

NINE WAYS TO TRAIN LIKE A REAL PRO

1. Always monitor your heart rate periodically, staying within your training range.
2. To lose weight and body fat, exercise at a lower intensity level for a longer duration.
3. If you're training for anaerobic capacity, work out at a medium pace, then increase your workouts to a high level of intensity for 30 to 60 seconds, then return to a moderate level. This is also called interval training or "fartlek."
4. To increase your cardiovascular power, exercise at a moderate pace, and vary the equipment or activity, duration, and intensity.
5. Don't get caught in an exercise rut. Vary activities or, if you prefer just one aerobic activity, alter the intensity one day, the duration the next. For instance, ride a hard mile one day, three easy miles the next.
6. Drink plenty of water before, during, and after your workout to replenish fluids lost through sweat. Beer or Java won't do the trick because they're both dehydrating rather than refreshing. The best replenisher is still H_2O.
7. If you find yourself getting tired before your workout time is over, slow the pace.
8. Give yourself a break! Only amateur athletes exercise every day rain or shine. Take off a day (or two or three a week) and avoid exercise burnout, fatigue, aches, and even insomnia.
9. Be patient. To see progress in the mirror, on the scale, or in the way your clothing fits, you have to commit to the program. Engage in at least 30 minutes of continuous aerobic exercise three times a week to burn fat and build cardiovascular strength. If you don't see progress, take an honest look at your workout schedule. Have you been a loyal, true-blue fan, or a fair weather friend? You won't get results without commitment, but once you're serious—wow!—you won't believe what you'll achieve.

THE SEARCH FOR A LEGITIMATE HEALTH CLUB

Remember that fancy fitness center you joined for the one-year, bargain-basement price—the one that folded six months later? Or the swank health club with the posh locker room and one stair climber? What about that new club near work where the aerobics instructor didn't know her biceps from her triceps?

It seems that everyone I know has a health club horror story. One friend was strong-armed at the door and nearly forced to join; another was conned about instructors' credentials.

Until recently, there were no governing bodies to boot out the less-than-professional clubs. But the American College of Sports Medicine has recently instituted a voluntary certification program that gives the ACSM stamp of approval to clubs that meet the grade in terms of equipment, fitness programs, safety, and ethical business practices. Hopefully, the voluntary program will set industry-wide standards that over time will weed out the imposters or substandard clubs.

ACSM's informative booklet: *ACSM Health/Fitness Facility Consumer Selection Guide* can help you in your search by outlining what to look for, important questions to ask, etc. For a free copy, send a stamped self-addressed envelope to ACSM, Box 1440, Indianapolis, IN 46206-1440. Meanwhile, here are a few helpful tips to keep in mind when searching for a club:

- Visit the club during the hours you would normally work out. If it feels overcrowded, dirty, shabby, or in general second-rate, the fitness program may be, too. Walk around and talk to members, eavesdrop on some aerobics classes, and check out the equipment-to-member ratio. (Lines for the stair climber, again, are a bad sign.)
- Find out how long the club has been in business. To avoid joining a fly-by-night, get a credit rating from the Better Business Bureau.
- Are the instructors certified (by the IDEA, American College of Sports Medicine, the Aerobics and Fitness Association of America or the Institute of Aerobics Research?) Are personal trainers available in the event you need assistance?
- Obtain a listing of classes; the club should offer a variety of aerobic classes on a schedule that fits yours.
- Check out the equipment. Is it state-of-the-art or a collection of broken-down and/or outdated rejects?
- Browse around the locker room and restrooms. If they don't pass the white-glove test, scoot!

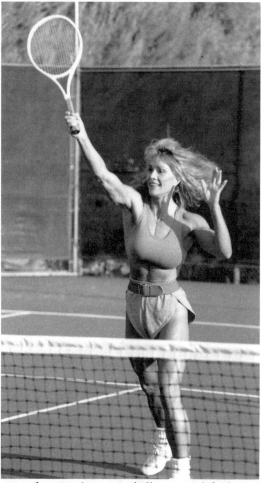

Don't let the sweat from sports such as tennis, racquetball, or squash fool you into thinking you're getting an aerobic workout. These sports involve too much stopping and starting—especially when I play. Much of my time goes to picking up the balls.

- Are the saunas and whirlpools coed or sex-segregated? You may feel more comfortable (and be safer) using women-only facilities.
- Is there a pool? Does it have Olympic-length lap lanes so you can swim without bumping into kids or senior "floaters?"
- Make sure the fee, hours, location, and class schedules match your budget and time restraints. Otherwise, you'll never use your membership.
- Never sign a lifetime membership. "Lifetime" often refers to the club's—not yours. With health clubs dying like flies, don't risk joining a club where the aerobics instructor runs out on you before your membership does.

AEROBIC COUNTDOWN

How well does your favorite aerobic activity build cardiovascular workout, upper and lower body strength? And is it a great calorie-burner, or just so-so? Use the following chart to find out— and if your favorite activity is low in one area, team it with one that fills in the gap for an exercise program that you enjoy, and which also covers all the fitness bases.

Don't forget, what you put into your workout is what you get out of it!

Key:

1. Cardiovascular workout
2. Upper body workout
3. Lower body workout
4. Calorie burn

Rating: Excellent=E; Average=A; Poor=P

Outdoor Sports

Backpacking: 1E/2A/3A/4A
Cycling: 1E/2A/3E/4E
Mountain Biking: 1E/2A/3E/4E
Rowing: 1E/2E/3P/4A
Hiking: 1E/2A/3A/4A
Speedwalking: 1E/2A/3E/4A
Horseback Riding: 1P/2A/3A/4A
Gymnastics: 1P/2E/3E/4P
In-line Skating: 1E/2A/3E/4E
Running: 1E/2P/3E/4E
Cross-Country Skiing: 1E/2E/3E/4E
Downhill Ski: 1P/2A/3E/4P
Swimming: 1E/2E/3E/4E
Rock Climbing: 1P/2E/3E/4A

Indoor Sports

Aerobics: 1E/2E/3E/4E
Ballet: 1P/2A/3E/4A
Boxing: 1E/2E/3A/4E
Step: 1E/2E/3E/4E
Yoga: 1P/2P/3P/4P

Exercise Machines

Upper Body: 1P/2E/3P/4E
Lower Body: 1P/2P/3E/4E
Step Machines: 1E/2P/3E/4E
Stair Climbers: 1E/2P/3E/4E
Treadmills: 1E/2A/3E/4E
Stationary Bikes: 1E/2P/3E/4E

Calorie Burn at a Glance (Per hour)

Backpacking: 600-825
Boxing: 525-600
Cycling: 625-850
Mountain Biking: 650-900
Speedwalking: about 450
Hiking: 525-700
Jogging (5.5 mph): about 650
Running (6.5 mph): about 750
In-Line Skating: 550-850
Vigorous Tennis: up to 600
Vigorous Handball: up to 600
Downhill Skiing: about 585
Cross-country Skiing: 650-900
Swimming: 350-530

GREAT EXERCISE VIDEOS

If you want to exercise at home, here are a few exercise videos I've put out to help you.

Step Aerobics

- *Step 'N Time,* by Cory Everson
- *Step Training Video,* by Cory Everson
- *Total Body Workout,* by Cory Everson

Weight Training/Conditioning

- *Cory Everson's: Lean Hips, Thighs and Buns* (slimming, toning and reshaping)
- *Cory Everson's: Beautiful Back Biceps and Abdominals* (slimming, toning and reshaping)
- *Cory Everson's: Shapely Chest, Triceps and Shoulders* (slimming, toning and reshaping)

Dance/Aerobic

- *Funky Bizness: Cardio Hip Hop Workout With Michelle LeMay*

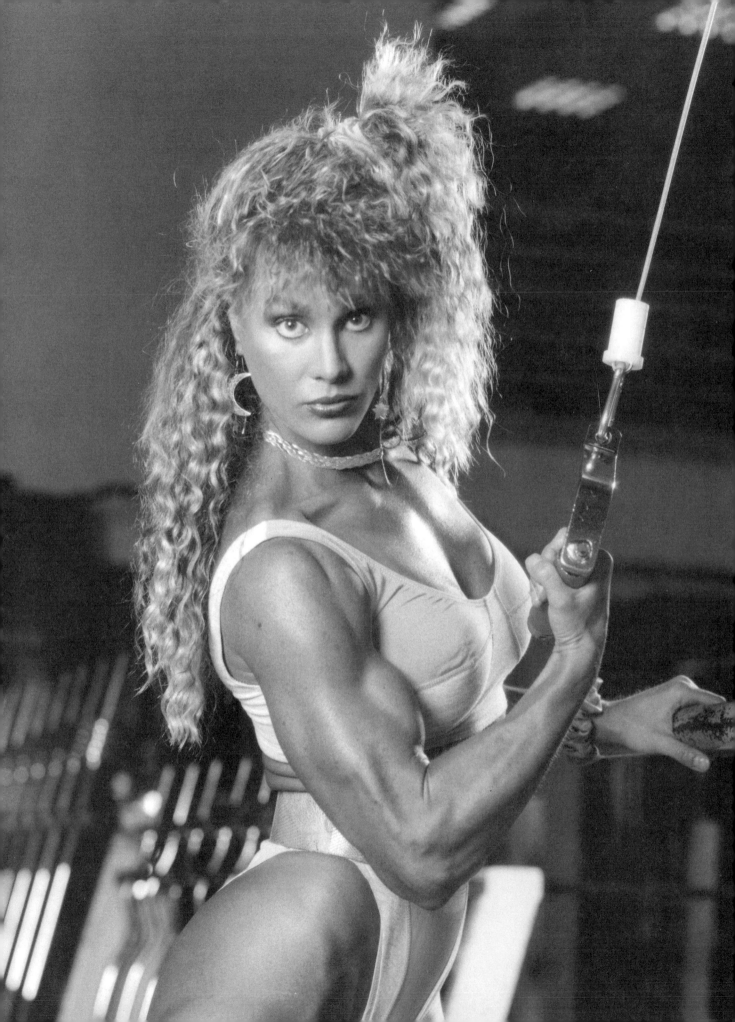

Eight
Aerobics, Too

We promised you workouts that would banish fat without boring you to death—and give you curves where you never knew they'd look so wonderful. So wriggle into your tights, lace up your shoes, and let's get ready to blast the fat with the following seven great aerobic workouts. It's now or never, ladies, so follow me!

For you speedwalking demons or wanna-bes, I'll show you a workout that leaves the fat in the dust—and fast.

Want total fun and fitness fun in the great outdoors? Try the "Outer Bounder" program, courtesy of Diana McNab, a former Olympic skier for Canada. This workout takes its cue from Mother Nature to deliver a guaranteed scenic sweat.

Prefer to exercise under cover? There's the Gym Workout for budding aerobettes. Under deep cover? Try the Homebody Workout.

Or put up yer dukes and find a full-length mirror. With our Knock 'Em Dead Shadowboxing Workout, your fat won't have a fighting chance.

Remember, if you're more than 20 pounds overweight, if you have medical problems, or are recuperating from a serious illness or injury, check with your physician before starting any exercise program.

LeMAY'S WAKE-UP YOUR METABOLISM WORKOUT

My favorite choreographer, Michelle LeMay, swears this workout routine will awaken your fat-burning furnace within.

This workout is based on principles of total body conditioning (developed by the Nike elite team), circuit training, and cross-country. It is designed for maximum benefit in minimum time. Not only will you maximize fat mobilization for weight loss, but you will also increase muscle tone, giving you a shapelier body and increasing your metabolism. Lastly, this workout has a built-in protection against hitting those frustrating plateaus. Just when your body starts getting accustomed to a particular exercise, we're going to change it and "shock your muscles." Not only will this keep you on track to a higher fitness level but it will also be a much more interesting way to battle the bulge. Most experts agree experts that people are more like likely to stick to a workout program they enjoy, so–have it your way. You choose the exercises.

Before beginning this program, I would like you to put pencil to paper. Review the list of cardio exercises below and make three lists for month 1, month 2, and month 3. Choose your three favorite cardiovascular exercises and place one on the top of each list. Then choose your next three favorite exercises and put them second on each list. If you enjoy enough of a variety of activities and have the equipment available, make your third choices and add them to the lists.

CARDIO EXERCISES TO CHOOSE FROM

Outdoor
Speed Walking
Jogging
Rollerskating
In-line Skating
Swimming
Stair Climbing (stadium)

Aerobics
Aerobics–high/low impact
Aerobics–low impact
Step Aerobics
Funk Aerobics
Boxercise
Water Aerobics

Machines and Apparatus
Treadmill
Stationary Bike
Step Machine
Stair Climber
Slide
Rower
Nordic Track

Example

Month 1	**Month 2**	**Month 3**
Walking	Stationary Biking	Step Aerobics
Rollerblade	Rowing Machine	Nordic Track
Funk Aerobics	Swimming	Slide

ELEMENTS OF THE WORKOUT

Warm-up and Cool-down

All workouts should begin with a short warm-up and end with a cool-down. Your warm-up is comprised of two sections: First, get the body warm, then do light stretching to prevent injury. Please note: Your warm-up stretch is not the best place to try to increase flexibility—save that for the cool-down when your muscles are nice and warm and more pliable.

Warm-up

1. 3–5 minutes—Get your blood flowing. Go for a brisk walk, hop on a bicycle, or even march in place pumping your arms.
2. 2–4 minutes—Light stretching for calves, hamstrings, quadriceps, hip flexors, and shoulders.

Cool-down

This is your time to relax, center yourself, and increase flexibility. Pat yourself on the back for a good workout, think positive thoughts, and focus on relaxing the muscle you're trying to stretch. Be patient while stretching. To increase flexibility, you need to hold each stretch 10–60 seconds.

Cardio-sections

This is where you will plug in the exercises on your lists. Start with month 1 and every time you see the word *cardio* appear on your workout, plug in one of the exercises you have chosen. Do this for three months, changing your type of cardio workout each month, and you've completed what Michelle calls one cycle. Once you have completed one cycle, you can repeat the cycles three more times to complete four cycles per year, or take one month off between cycles and end up with a total of three cycles per year.

INTERVALS

Interval training is a great way to push yourself to a higher fitness level. It involves short bouts of intense exercise with active recovery periods. This allows you to work at higher intensities than you would have been able to work at without that recovery period.

If you are just beginning this program, work in the mid to upper part of your THR range for the short, intense bouts, and the lower range for your active recovery. If you're an athlete and desire an increase in physical performance, you can actually push more in the short, intense bouts (utilizing your anaerobic system), and work in your low to mid THR range during your active recovery periods.

Active Recovery Segments

Continue to do your cardio exercise; however, slow your pace a bit.

Resistance Segments

These exercises can be done with weights, rubber bands, machinery, or using your own body weight to create the resistance. There are hundreds of different resistence exercises to do, (refer to chapter 9, "Weight-training Your Way to a More Beautiful Body," as well as *Cory Everson's Workout,* Perigee Books. Most important, choose resistance exercises where your head remains above the heart. Also, be sure to work all antagonistic muscles equally. Work at your own pace. For example:

Beginniers—Bicep curls with light dumbbells
Intermediates—Increase the intensity by adding a squat
Advanced or Competitive athletes—Add the squat and increase the weight.

The following is a list of just some of the equipment and movements you can use for the resistance sections of the workouts that follow.

EQUIPMENT	MOVEMENTS
Dumbbells	Bicep Curls
Bodybars	Overhead Tricep Extension
Elastic tubing	Overhead Press
Hydrafitness equipment	Lateral Raises
	Squats
	Lunges
	Plies

DAY ONE (55-MINUTE WORKOUT)

- 4–7 minute warm-up and stretch
- 20 minutes cardio (insert your cardio choices)
- 20 minutes interval (4 minutes cardio recovery, 1 minute resistance)
- 8–12 minute cool-down/stretch

DAY TWO (40–MINUTE WORKOUT)

- 4–7 minute warm-up
- 25 minute cardio (insert your choices)
- 8–12 minute cool-down

DAY THREE (45 MINUTES)

- 4–7 minute warm-up
- 20 minute cardio (insert your choices)
- 10 minute interval (60 seconds resistance, 90 seconds cardio recovery)
- 8–12 minute cool-down

BEGINNERS BE SMART

I know your motivation level is high right now. You took your first step by buying this book. Now it's time to put all your new knowledge into action! Be smart, listen to your body! Start off slow and gradually increase at a comfortable pace. For example, Day One includes 20 minutes of straight cardio plus 20 minutes of interval training. Start with 10 minutes of cardio and 10 minutes of interval training, and gradually increase as you become more fit.

CORY'S SPEED DEMON WORKOUT (FIVE DAYS, 40–60 MINUTES A DAY)

Ladies, tie your laces. With this workout you'll literally speedwalk away your excess fat in a few months. Combine it with a good stretching program, add weight training three times a week, and you're on the high road to fitness.

As you walk, here are a few speedwalking moves you can use to work your upper body and increase caloric expenditure.

- Windmills: As you walk, move your arms as if you are doing the backstroke.
- Sleepwalkers: Just like it sounds. Extend your arms as if you're trying to reach something in front of you.
- Reach and pull.

DAY ONE

- 3 mile walk (13- to 14-minute a mile pace)
- 1 mile easy walking with Moves described above
- ½ mile cool-down
- 10 minutes stretching

DAY TWO

- 2 minutes easy walking with Moves
- 2-mile speedwalk
- ½ mile cool-down
- 10 minutes stretching

DAY THREE

- 20 minutes upper body weight training
- 2 mile speed walk
- ½ mile cool-down

DAY FOUR

- 4-mile speedwalk
- half mile cool-down
- 10 minutes stretching

DAY FIVE

- 20 minutes total body weight training
- 1 mile easy walk with Moves
- ½-mile cool-down

HOMEBODY WORKOUT (THREE DAYS, 45–75 MINUTES A WEEK)

- dumbbells
- bench
- bar

For those who don't live near a gym or prefer to exercise at home, this workout is a cheap sweat that burns fat without investing in anything but time and energy. All you'll need is dumbbells, a bench, and a bar. Finally! A workout studio where you can dress like a slob or even exercise in your undies.

DAY ONE

- 30-minutes speedwalk OR 20-minute hike OR 25-minute jog OR 30-minute cycle
- 15–20 minutes weight training (total body)
- 10 minutes stretching

DAY TWO

- 45–60 minutes hiking OR 30–40 minutes walking OR 20 minutes bench or stair stepping
- 15–20 minutes upper body weight training
- 10 minutes stretching

DAY THREE

- 30 minutes cycling OR 20 minutes hiking OR 30 minutes jogging OR 45 minutes walking
- 15–20 minutes total body weight training
- 10 minutes stretching

HEALTH CLUB WORKOUT (FOUR DAYS, 45–90 MINUTES A DAY)

You love the gym so much you have underwear with the names of the week on them—and matching tights. Here's a weekly workout for those of you who prefer the company of others and instruction afforded by a group workout with an instructor as opposed to solitary sweats.

This workout combines aerobic dance class routines with exercise machines, free weights, and body-sculpting regimens—the best from your local gym.

DAY ONE

- 45 minutes aerobics or bench aerobics
- 15 minutes upper body weight training
- 10 minutes stretching

DAY TWO

- 20 minutes rowing OR 20 minutes stair climbing OR 30 minutes on treadmill OR 30 minutes on exercise cycle. (Feel like a kid in a candy store? Me, too! Just pick your favorites and you're all set!)
- 15 minutes lower body weight training
- 10 minutes stretching

DAY THREE

- 45–60 minutes aerobics and 15 minutes upper body strengthening OR
- 60 minutes bench aerobics
- 10 minutes stretching

DAY FOUR

- 30 minutes total-body circuit training OR 20 minutes rowing OR 30 minutes cycling OR 20 minutes stair climbing
- 10 minutes stretching

LEAN MACHINE WORKOUT (FIVE DAYS, 45–60 MINUTES PER DAY)

You'd rather walk a treadmill than a trail, climb a stair climber than a mountain, and ride the sort of bicycle that goes nowhere fast. The perfect workout for women who prefer to exercise under cover—or for outdoor enthusiasts grounded by bad weather.

DAY ONE

- 30 minutes treadmill walking, middle-range intensity
- 5 minute cool-down
- 10 minutes stretching

DAY TWO

- 20 minutes on exercise bicycle
- 5 minute cool-down
- 10 minutes stretching
- 10 minutes upper body weight training

DAY THREE

- 30 minutes stair climbing on your favorite hill program, middle-range intensity
- 5 minute cool-down
- 10 minutes stretching

DAY FOUR

- 20 minutes on treadmill, alternating 7 minutes middle range pace with 1-minute high range, then back to middle range
- 5 minute cool-down
- 10 minutes stretching
- 20 minutes lower body weight training

DAY FIVE

- 15 minutes on stair climber—flat program
- 15 minutes on treadmill, medium range
- 5 minute cool-down
- 10 minutes stretching

OUTER BOUNDER WORKOUT (FIVE DAYS, 45–70 MINUTES A DAY)

If nature is your favorite gym, you'll love this workout, which gets you in the great outdoors enough to qualify for permanent Sierra Club status. You total purists can even do the stretching exercises and weight-training stuff outdoors.

Ready to rip, roll, ride, or skate? Good! We're outa here!

DAY ONE

- 50 minutes hiking or speedwalking (find a nice, steep hill and go for it)
- 10 minutes stretching

DAY TWO

- 40 minutes mountain biking, cycling, or in-line skating
- 20 minutes upper body weight training
- 10 minutes stretching

DAY THREE

- 50 minutes in-line skating or cross-country skiing
- 10 minutes stretching

DAY FOUR

- 30 minutes trail jogging
- 20 minutes upper body weight training
- 10 minutes stretching

DAY FIVE

Play day! Enjoy your favorite aerobic sport for an entire hour—or longer if you have the time and energy. Turn it into interval training by pushing moderately hard for 15 minutes, then crank into high gear for a minute or so and slip back to a moderate pace. Don't neglect your stretching exercises before you go!

KNOCK 'EM DEAD WORKOUT (THREE TIMES A WEEK, 45–60 MINUTES)

Put up your dukes; your fat won't have a fighting chance with this boxing workout that borrows aerobic moves from the Big Ring. From lunging to shadowboxing, the boxing workout (which you do alone in front of a mirror) uses all the major muscle groups for a rigorous bout. Even better, with this form of boxing, you're always the uncontested winner. So knock yourself out.

BASIC WORKOUT

- 10 minutes stretching
- 1½ minutes jumping rope; rest, and repeat
- 5 rounds of shadowboxing, each round lasting 1½ minutes each with 1-minute rests in between. Face the mirror and mix and match the following moves to work up a sweat:

1. Jab: Punch with your left arm, twisting it so your hand is parallel to the ground

2. Straight Right: Punch with your right arm, twist it so your hand is parallel to the ground, aiming for chin or higher in the mirror.

3. Left Hook: Raising your right elbow, bend arms at right angle, parallel to ground; shift weight to left foot and swing arm across face as if you were going to strike your opponent on the side of his chin.

4. Uppercut: Crouching slightly with bent knees, bring your right hand to your chest, with your arm bent. Jab as if you were hitting your opponent under the nose. Pivot on your right foot and keep your left foot firmly planted.

TWENTY-TWO WAYS TO FALL IN LOVE WITH EXERCISE

1. Make It a Habit

Whoever said use it or lose it wasn't kidding. Studies show that once you stop working out, you could lose more than half of your muscular fitness in about three months. Aerobic capacity may take even less time to evaporate—as little as a month or two if you go from a rigorous schedule to nothing.

2. Try It by Twilight

Exercise around 5 P.M. and you'll sleep like a baby. Studies show early evening exercise helps you wind down for bedtime. Don't exercise too late, however, or it could overenergize you so you're up all night.

3. Get Aerobic for at Least 20–30 Minutes Three Times a Week

Exercise for at least 30 minutes at least three times a week and check your pulse to make sure you're at the pace that's safe for you. Running, jogging, swimming, cycling, hiking, aerobic dance, cross-country skiing, speedskating, speed walking—anything that gives your pulse a rise and works up a sweat. If you aren't perspiring, it isn't aerobic, so pick up the pace. Studies show that the rate at which you burn fat increases after about 20 minutes and jumps to 70 percent after that. The moral of the story? Thirty minutes is essential; 45 minutes to an hour is even better.

4. Cool It!

Sweat means you're losing water your body would otherwise use to keep you healthfully hydrated. To maintain your cool, especially when exercising during hot summer months, drink whenever you're thirsty and tank up before a workout with as much as you can drink, preferably a quart of water. To find out how much water you typically lose, weigh yourself before and right after a workout and drink enough to account for sweat losses and then some. If you've lost a pound in one hour, you've lost one pint, or two cups of sweat, so drink up accordingly. Water is best, but carbonated soda is OK to drink before workouts. New studies show the bubbles have no deleterious effects on performance on your stomach. As far as post-workout, water is better than soda pop because the bubbles in soda pop can create a sense of fullness so you stop drinking before completely replenishing your fluids.

To rapidly replace sweat losses, try sports drinks; their electrolyte content puts liquids back in you pronto—even faster than water.

While cold water keeps you slightly cooler than warm, it has to be inside you to work. While wetting may feel refreshing, it has no measurable effect on your body's core temperature.

5. Get Out of the Rut With Cross-training

Why risk exercise boredom by doing the same ole' workout day in and day out. Try aerobic dance one day, cycling the next, jogging another day, hiking in the mountains or rollerblading by the beach another day. Although calorie differences may vary slightly, the important thing is to get out there and just do it—whatever you feel like doing that day.

6. Plan a Fitness Break

Job got you tied to your desk with no time to exercise? Use your vacation time to jump-start a new exercise program. Try a fitness-oriented spa (see Chapter 9 for the most aerobic-minded spas), or plan an active adventure travel or fitness-type vacation, like a cycling vacation. Or go trekking someplace high, like the Colorado Rockies or Nepal, or learn a new sport like rock climbing, tennis, sea kayaking—anything that requires you to move it.

7. Get High

We're talking about altitude. Research shows you burn nearly a third more calories when exercising at high altitudes over 14,000 feet because your body's metabolic mechanisms shift because of the lack of oxygen.

8. Rise and Aerobicize

I know—we just told you to exercise in the evening. But if your hectic lifestyle has you going from dawn to dusk, exercise first thing in the morning so you're sure to fit it in. If you wait until you return home, the gym may be closed, it may be too dark outside, or you may be too tired. Studies show those who exercise in the morning are most likely to be exercising a year down the road; only half of those who exercise at mid-day continue longterm. Only one in four who exercises in the evening stick with it. Apparently, the later it gets, the more time you have to come up with excuses not to exercise. I know this for a fact, as I have never been one to stick with a regular evening workout.

9. Twist and Shout

Nothing will increase your pace like moving to music. Not only does music lower your perception of pain and fatigue, but if it's really a grooving tempo, you may find yourself jogging or cycling faster just to keep up with the music. Music also tends to create steady, rhythmic motion so you can better regulate your breathing and establish a good pace.

The best place for headsets or music is in the gym. Outdoors, some sports that lend themselves to headsets are jogging, speedwalking, and hiking—but not rollerblading or cycling because music is a dangerous distraction in traffic. Indoors or out, keep the volume down to a comfortable level; loud music blasting in your eardrums over just a few weeks can mean irreparable hearing loss.

10. Chill Out

Those of you who live in areas where things freeze in the winter know what happens when you exercise outdoors: you lose weight because your body has to warm you against the elements. Although we're not recommending that you tropical or desert dwellers exercise in walk-in freezers, a ski trip could be just the temporary jump-start your body needs to shed a few pounds.

11 . . . Or Heat Up Your Workout

You'll also burn more calories when exercising in hot, humid weather because your body has to expend more to cool you. Be careful in both cases; really cold weather carries the risk of hypothermia while aerobic exercise in extremely hot temps can invite sunstroke or dehydration.

12. Lift and Lose

Studies show that women who lift weights and engage in aerobic exercise lose more fat than those who engage only in aerobic activity. This is because weight lifting builds muscle, which weighs more than fat. According to researchers at Emory University in Atlanta, women who included circuit weight training in their weight loss programs lost 13 percent more fat than those who just did aerobics; they also maintained more muscles. Nothing dumb about dumbbells.

13. Go for the Long Haul—Not the Quick Burn

You'll burn more calories exercising at a slow or moderate rate for an hour than sprinting or racing for 20 minutes, according to research at the San Diego State University. Rather than running or cycling up a steep hill and getting exhausted in less than a half hour, take a longer, more gentle ride and you'll not only burn more calories but feel more relaxed and refreshed.

14. Time It Right to Slim Down

Are you more than 30 percent over your ideal weight? Then exercise before a meal and you'll burn calories. Conversely, if you're less than 30 percent above your ideal weight, exercise after eating.

15. Climb On

You know those steps that lead up to your 14th floor office? Take them instead of the elevator and you'll be that much closer to your ideal weight. In fact, you can make a daily workout on the fire escape if you're really desperate.

16. Join a Health Club

Nothing helps you establish a regular exercise program like belonging to a gym; even I belong to one, though I have a workout room at home.

The camaraderie, exercise options, including a range of machines and trainers who can assist you, make for a perfect learning environment. Plus you'll make new fitness friends, who can encourage and motivate you to stay aerobic.

The money your fork out may well be the best bucks you ever spend—even if you normally exercise outdoors, a health club is good aerobic insurance against bad weather, when you may be tempted to skip working out because it's raining, snowing, too hot, too cold, or too dark.

17. Workouts on the Road

A growing number of hotels are offering guests exercise options—from full-fledged health clubs down to closet-sized cubes with treadmill or exercise bike. Maintaining a regular exercise program on the road will keep you invigorated, regulate your appetite in the face of two-hour business lunches, and provide stamina for surviving endless board meetings. It can also help combat jet lag; exercising in natural light on arrival can "jog" your internal clock to local time. Ask the hotel receptionist for a jogging or biking map. If your hotel lacks exercise facilities, ask the receptionist about local health clubs where, for a small fee, you can "join" for a day or two, use fitness equipment, and even take classes. If your travels take you to the boonies where clubs and gyms are miles away, tuck a jump rope into your suitcase and exercise right in your hotel room.

18. Got That Draggin' Feeling?

It may indicate an iron deficiency. If you feel like it's too much to even walk across the room—that heavy legs syndrome—ask your doctor to test you for anemia. Studies show that women who were iron deficient used less oxygen during exercise and thus tended to accumulate more lactic acid—the substance that makes muscles feel heavy and achy.

19. Pregnant or Planning to Be?

Contrary to old wives' tales, being pregnant doesn't mean you necessarily must give up your workout, although if you're a couch potato this is no time to start training for a marathon. Provided you already exercise regularly, you may be able to keep up a modified workout up to the date of delivery. Check with your physician—you may be pleasantly surprised.

20. Get a Checkup First

If you're obese, more than 20 percent overweight, or recovering from a serious illness, surgery, or injury, talk to your doctor before beginning any exercise program. Although exercise is often just what the doctor ordered, better safe than sorry.

21. Get an Exercise Buddy

If you tend to loose interest in exercise after a few weeks, find an exercise buddy to keep you on track.

Someone at your level of fitness can be just the "nudge" you need to keep going. And times flies when you're having fun, so join a walking, hiking, or cycling club that holds weekly outings and you'll really look forward to your workouts!

22. Don't Give Up—Ever

Rome wasn't built in a day, so don't get discouraged if after a week or so you haven't lost any inches or pounds. Give yourself at least a month for results to show. If you follow your nutrition and exercise program, the results will show and you won't be the only one who notices. That's a promise.

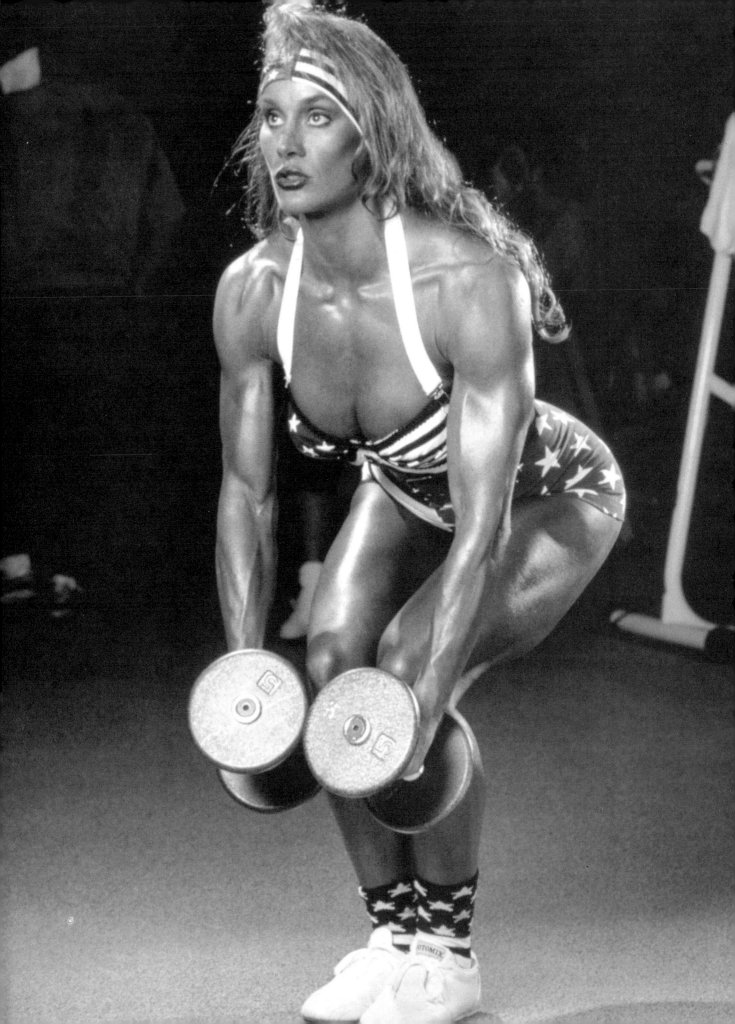

Nine

Weight Training Your Way to a More Beautiful Body

Weight training is a precise science. Train the wrong way and you'll waste a lot of time. But train the right way using the right muscles and most importantly, your brain, and you can maximize your curves, minimize your bulges, and make the most of your inherited attributes.

As we mentioned earlier, many women fear weight training will put hair on their chests and bulge their biceps.

Fat chance! Take it from me—building bulging muscles is a fulltime job requiring four- to six-hour daily workouts in addition to a super high-protein diet and the right genetic makeup. You couldn't do that on this program if you slept with your barbells. Besides, our goal is not a body like Arnold's (sorry!), but feminine muscles that convey a sense of strength without turning you into Brunhilda.

How much time will this take? Sit down. How does 90 minutes a week sound, divided into three 30-minute sessions? It will probably take you longer to read this chapter than complete an entire week's worth of weight training, although I strongly recommend you read it before lifting so much as a three-pound weight.

ELEVEN REASONS WHY YOU SHOULD WEIGHT TRAIN

The weight of evidence has become too heavy to ignore. Weight training accomplishes all this and more:

1. It builds muscle that burns fat so you lose weight faster. Muscles are active tissues that burn calories to maintain themselves. Most fat is inert and good only to insulate us in very cold weather, like the North Pole. (Just ask Santa.)

2. It decreases your risk of developing heart disease.

3. It helps fend off high blood pressure.

4. It helps prevent adult-onset diabetes.

5. It minimizes your chances of developing coronary heart disease in later years.

6. It builds stronger bones to help protect you against osteoporosis, which is not a disease that afflicts only grannies. Boomers are vulnerable, too, and new studies show that younger women in their thirties, especially Caucasian women with slight builds, may get osteoporosis before they get their first gray hair if their diets lack calcium, or if they drink and/or smoke to excess and don't exercise regularly.

(For free information on osteoporosis, send a large, self-addressed stamped envelope to the National Osteoporosis Foundation, Box A, 1150 17th St., NW, Suite 500, Washington, DC 20036.)

7. It helps ease tension and stress which can be a contributing factor in diseases ranging from migraines to cancer. With weight training, you can lift your troubles away.

8. It increases your level of confidence. Remember when Charles Atlas convinced millions of men to build big muscles so other guys wouldn't kick sand in their faces? When you look strong physically, you feel strong mentally and emotionally, too—and also convey a sense of inner strength.

9. It's simple to learn.

10. It can be very inexpensive and performed at home with cheap dumbbells.

11. It's downright sexy. Muscles are very much in vogue these days; just ask Madonna or check out the fashion magazines. Gone are the Twiggy clones with their skinny little arms and barely-there butts. Even the thinnest models today have pretty, feminine biceps and curves. That's the look we're shooting for here—not gigantic, bulging muscles but shapely ones as in Janet Jackson, Cher, Heather Locklear, Raquel Welsh, Jane Fonda, Demi Moore . . .

GYMS ARE FUN

Where to work out? It's your choice. A health club offers the most versatility in terms of weight training, and the good ones have certified exercise instructors on hand to answer questions and make sure you're following a safe and effective training program. Many gyms offer personalized trainers for one-on-one advice. Gyms are a great way to get out of the house or office. And if you're new to the fitness scene, you can make new exercise buddies, pick their brains for advice, and get into the swing of things faster.

Finally, may I offer a word of support to you novices out there who are a little shy about going to a gym alone? Some of the nicest people in the world work out in gyms and I should know, having spent a large part of my life in them. So don't be intimidated by all that Lycra. Find a gym that meets the qualifications we explained in Chapter 8 and after a few visits, it'll feel like a second home. If it doesn't, find another gym.

On the other hand, if you're more of a 9 to 9er than a 9 to 5er and gym schedules are tough to squeeze into, or you just don't have the bucks to join, there are still lots of training options. A home gym is a great alternative that can consist of a collection of free weights and barbells—definitely the budget way to go and the most common. Some people find free weights unwieldy and are afraid they'll drop them on themselves or throw their backs out, but there's still another option.

The new generation of light-weight, space-saving machines means you don't need a reinforced floor or separate room to house them. Instead of the heavy metal plates of yesteryear, today's machines are fitted with superstrong rubber bands, hydraulic pistons, or cables attached to reels which provide resistance. Whatever the cost, at-home machines offer convenience and a wide range of exercises.

But buyer beware: Deluxe versions can set you back a few thousand dollars while cheap-o versions ($150 or less) are usually a complete waste of money. Not only are they clunky and cumbersome, but they can break down if you breathe on them. You're far better off investing in an inexpensive collection of dumbbells, which is all you'll need for the body sculpting workout we describe in this chapter. Start with three, five, or eight pounds and work up to 10 to 15 pounds.

GETTING STARTED

Where to begin? If you're new to weight training, our Strength and Body Sculpting Workout is just what you need to break in safely and easily—and I'll be holding your hand the entire way. (Holding the weights is up to you!)

With weight training, correct form and technique are both essential for results to show. Lift the wrong way or too much and you could wind up wasting a lot of time recuperating from sore muscles or injuries. Soreness that lasts longer than 72 hours may signal a strain, which means you should put off training that uses those muscles. If the soreness continues, you should see a physician.

Naturally, you'll want to combine your weight-training program with a diet high in complex carbs and low in fat (see the first five chapters), plus a good aerobics program (see Chapters 7–8).

BODY TRAINING LINGO

Weight training, like any sport, has its own vocabulary. Here are a few key terms to help you find your way around the gym—and so you don't slap the first guy who comments on your nice "set."

- Set: A group of exercises (10 bicep curls, for example)—see what we mean?
- Rep: Lifting a weight once is called a "rep," short for repetition.
- Tension: The amount of force exerted by a muscle when it contracts.
- Intensity: Your level of effort. The amount of weight you use relative to your absolute maximum. If you're lifting five pounds and your absolute maximum is 10, you're working at 50 percent intensity.
- Agility: The ability to change direction and speed of movement quickly.
- Proportion: Balanced muscle development.
- Stretching: Moving your limbs to a point where there's a slight discomfort in muscle and

supporting connective tissues. Holding this point is called static stretching.

- Flexion: Moving your arm, leg, or body from its normal anatomical position so that your muscle insertion moves closer to its origin. (As in flexing your biceps.)
- Extension: Moving your arm, leg, or body back to normal position after going through flexion. (Straightening your arm back to its normal position after flexing a bicep.)
- Contraction: Another name for muscle shortening. Also called "positive exercise."
- Pronation: Turning your palms down or your ankles in.
- Aerobic: Exercise where oxygen is used to produce energy. Nonstop exercise for at least 20 minutes to elevate your heart rate to 60–80 percent of your maximum (speedwalking, jogging, cross-country skiing, etc.).
- Anaerobic (without oxygen): Exercise that does not significantly increase your lung power or endurance (leisurely walking or cycling, power lifting), or very intense exercise, like sprinting, when the muscles are performing in the absence of oxygen.
- Endurance: Your "wind," or heart and lung capacity. Developed primarily through aerobic workouts.
- Fartlek: Also called interval training, or alternating sessions of power exercise with endurance exercise or rest. (It is not to be mistaken for intestinal flatulence)
- LSD workouts: No, it's not what it sounds like. It stands for "Long, Slow, Distance" workouts to burn fat and develop cardiovascular strength (long-distance cycling, slow jogging, in-line skating, etc.).
- Symmetry: Developing your muscles so your parts "match."
- PRE: (Progressive resistance exercise) Progressively increasing the amount of resistance or weight you use on an exercise.
- Working to failure: Performing reps until you reach total fatigue on the worked muscles!
- Spot toning: Concentrating on one area of your body to increase muscle tone; for instance, doing crunches to increase muscle tone in your abdominals.
- Spot reduction: Bogus theory that you can reduce body fat in one area of your body by exercising that particular part ad nauseum. For instance, doing endless leg lifts to trim thunderthighs. Wishful thinking, but no cigar.
- Rest period: The time between your workouts. Highly recommended to avoid overtraining. Remember—even God rested on the seventh day.
- Warm-up: Calisthenics and sustained activity elevates core body temperature before your workout, lubricates the joints, and increases blood flow to the muscles.
- Cool-down period: Very light movement and stretching following your exercise to bring your heart rate back down to normal and prevent blood from pooling in your legs, which could cause dizziness.
- Overtraining: Overdoing your exercise program, which can lead to chronic fatigue, physical, and mental burn-out and even (just what you need at a time like this!) insomnia.
- Split workouts: An exercise program where you work your upper body one day and your lower body the next training day, or working different body parts on different days.
- Circuit training: A series of exercises with little or no rest. Informally known as a "killer workout." It makes your weight workout more aerobic and burns more fat.
- Cycle workouts: Rotating workouts to stress intensity or volume, and, at other times, toning.
- Barbell: The shaft connecting weight plates and collars. A regular bar with collars weighs about 20 pounds.

- Free weights: Small, hand-held dumbbells that come in weights ranging from about three pounds to ten pounds.
- Spotters: Guardian angels who assist you during a workout. Often used for gymnastic-type moves involving aerial moves. (Don't worry—all the moves in my workout are grounded.) We won't be getting anywhere near the sort of weight that requires a spotter.
- Buffed: Looking great with muscle tone and definition; our end goal.

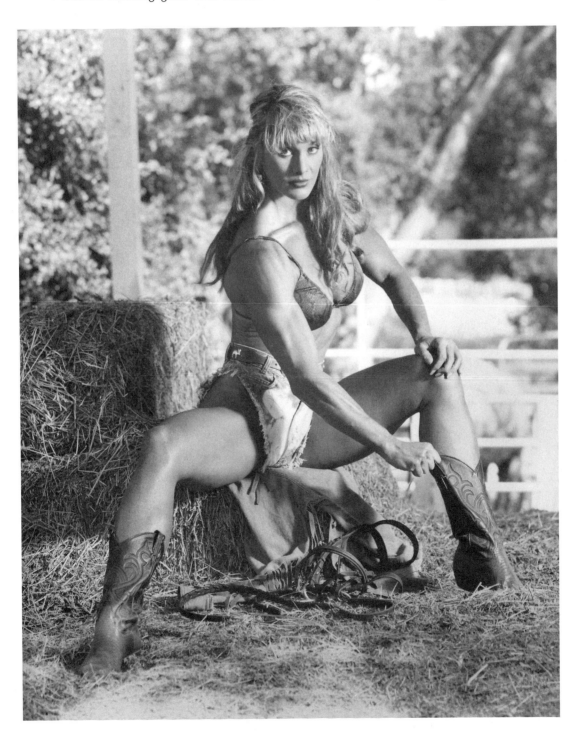

NITTY-GRITTIES

In weight training, form is function. How you lift is far more important than how much you lift. Pretty, feminine muscles come from lifting lighter weights for higher repetitions—even I don't lift anything heavier than 15 pounds these days. If you're a novice, you'll start out with three- or five-pound dumbbells and gradually progress to 15 pounds, plus or minus (unless you're interested in building serious muscle), working out for about 30 minutes on three alternating days: for instance, Monday-Wednesday-Friday or Tuesday-Thursday-Saturday. Stay on this introductory program for at least three weeks before trying anything more demanding or adding more weight.

Before you pick up that dumbbell, what comes first? Right! Stretching. If you skimmed over that section in Chapter 6, go back and read it very carefully. After your workout, cool down by walking, stretching, or cycling.

For your weight-training workout, choose one to three different exercises for each group of muscles. For your upper body, repeat each of those three exercises 10 to 20 times; these are called "reps" for repetition. Repeat each set of exercises three times, or do three "sets." To work your lower body, do three "sets" of exercises consisting of 10 to 30 "reps" of one to three different exercises. Here's how a typical progression from week one through week three might look:

WEEK ONE: 3 alternate days; about 20–30 minutes

- 1 set, using 2 exercises per body part
- 10 reps for upper body exercises
- 10 for lower body exercises

WEEK TWO: 3 alternate days; 30 minutes

- 2 sets of each exercise, using 2 exercises per body part
- 10 reps for upper body
- 15 reps for lower body

WEEK THREE: 3 alternate days; 30 minutes

- 2 sets of each exercise, using 2 exercises per body part
- 12 reps for upper body
- 20 reps for lower body

GENERAL WEIGHT-LIFTING GUIDELINES

After three weeks, gradually increase your workout weight, exercises, and sets. There's no magic formula—your body will set the upper limits and tell you when you need to add weight to create more resistance. Here are some general guidelines before we get started:

1. To develop only strength, do 1–5 repetitions of heavier weights. Try to use a weight which is heavy enough so that it is *difficult* to get more than 5 or 6 reps. If you get 8 or 9 reps, it is too light. Take longer rests between sets.
2. To build endurance, 20–50 reps with shorter rest between sets.

3. Use a slow, steady technique. To build strength, endurance, and lose body fat, do 10–20 reps for upper body and 10–30 reps for the lower body, with medium rests between sets.

4. Rest between sets—about 30–60 seconds is best to burn fat and build muscle. (Unless you're doing circuit training, in which case you don't rest at all between sets.)

5. Work big muscles before little muscles, since the larger muscle groups will take longer to tire.

6. Never hold your breath while weight training. Breathe in while lowering weights and exhale when you lift.

7. Be disciplined. Stick to your program. Envision yourself shapelier.

8. Have patience. Give yourself at least three months for results to show.

9. And our cardinal rule: Never start an exercise program without your doctor's consent, especially if you're overweight or recovering from an illness or injury.

Special tips if you're over thirty-five:

- Spend more time warming up and cooling down
- Don't use as much weight
- Skip the squats (see my list of favorite 18 below) and substitute another exercise

TIMING YOUR WORKOUTS (WORKOUT FREQUENCY)

Consistency and commitment—not dumbbells—are what build muscles. If you work out really hard only once a month, you won't make any progress because your workout frequency will be too low. On the other hand, if you go overboard and overtrain, you won't progress because your muscles won't have time to recover.

For best results, you must work out enough to force a response. This is called workout intensity. If you work out with the right frequency but use too little weight, you won't make headway. A combination of the right weights plus the right frequency equals success.

Structure your workout in one of two ways. You can either work your entire body during each workout, or do split workouts, working your upper body one day and your lower body on the next workout day. Either way, you'll want to alternate workout days and weight train no more than three or four days a week.

MY FAVORITE EIGHTEEN EXERCISES

There are more weight-training moves than we could possible describe in this chapter. If you want a variety of workouts and more exercises, my previous book *Cory Everson's Workout* (1991, Perigee Books), provides more than 30 different workouts broken down into specific sports activities, including specific workouts for knee and shoulder rehabilitation.

Meanwhile, let's look at a few new workouts I've developed for you that incorporate my 18 favorite body-sculpting and strengthening moves. Whether you're a beginner or an advanced weight trainer, they're guaranteed to bring out those curves. Feel free to mix and match them for your individual workout.

Five for Great Legs

1. SQUAT (without barbell for beginners, with barbell for intermediate and advanced): Strengthens front of thigh, rear of thigh, and buttocks.

A. Stand with a barbell across the back of your trapezius muscles. Use a grip (wide or narrow) on the bar that is most comfortable for you.

B. Position your legs where your feet are at least shoulder-width apart, preferably about 3–4 inches wider than your shoulders. Your feet should not point straight ahead but angle outward at a 45-degree angle.

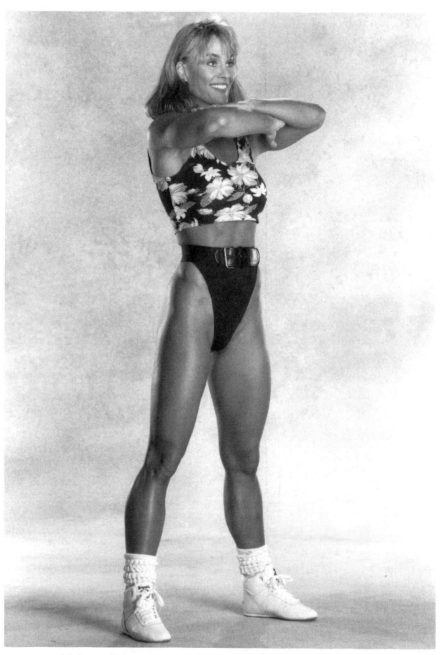

Never squat so your thighs are below parallel to the ground. As you progress, you can add weight.

C. Keep your back straight, eyes forward, and squat down to a point where the tops of your thighs are parallel with the floor. Make sure as you go down and come up that your knees are always in the same direct line as your feet.

D. Descend slowly. You can use a 2–3 inch block under your heels when you squat. With your heels elevated, you can keep your back more upright, which in turn puts more stress on your thighs instead of on your back and gluteus (butt, remember?).

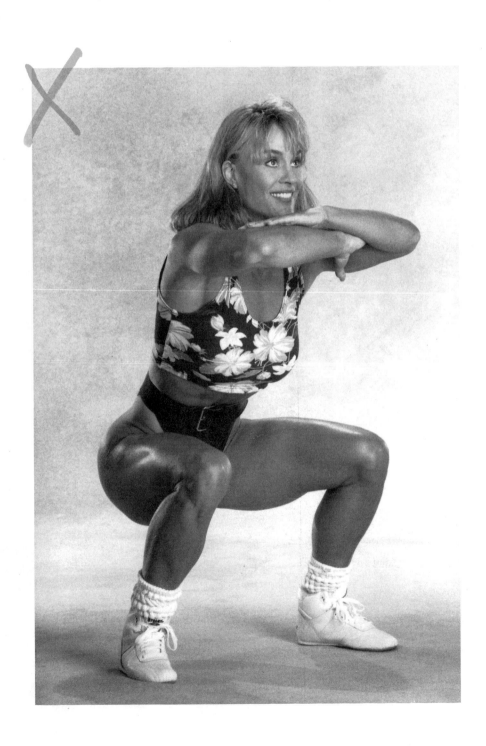

2. LEG EXTENSION: Sculpts and strengthens front of thigh.

A. Sit on a special quad-extension machine with your back pressed against the pad and your ankles under rollers.

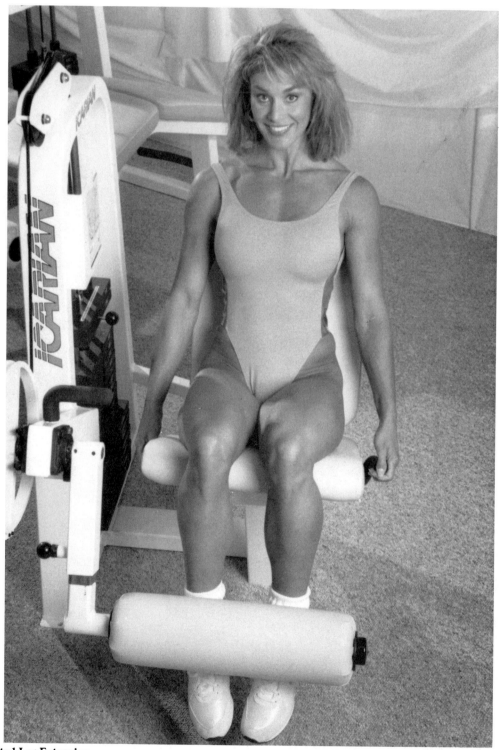

Seated Leg Extension

B. Straighten legs, lifting rollers to hip height and maintaining a slightly flexed position at the top. Squeeze those muscles and feel them tighten.

C. Return to starting position and repeat.

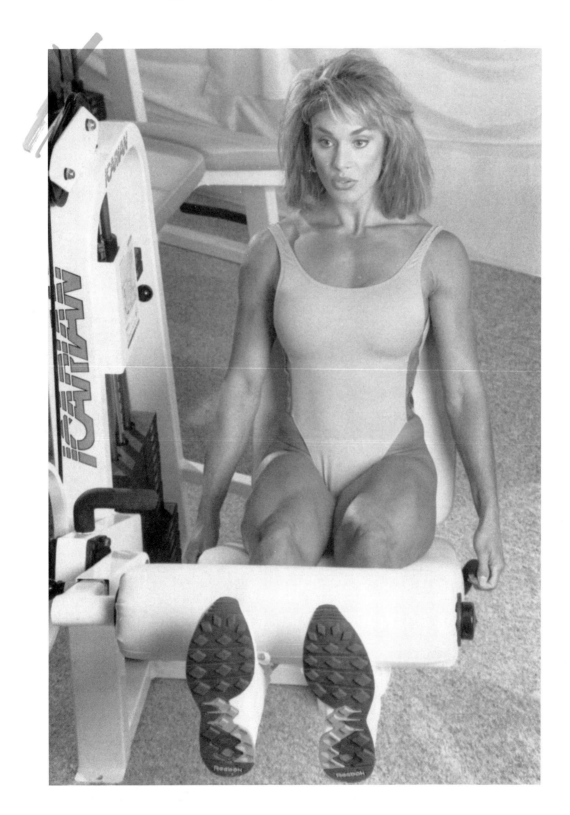

3. LEG CURL: Sculpts and strengthens rear of thigh, or hamstrings group.

A. Lie face down on the bench of a leg-curl machine, with head and spine in a straight line, legs extended and heels under rollers.

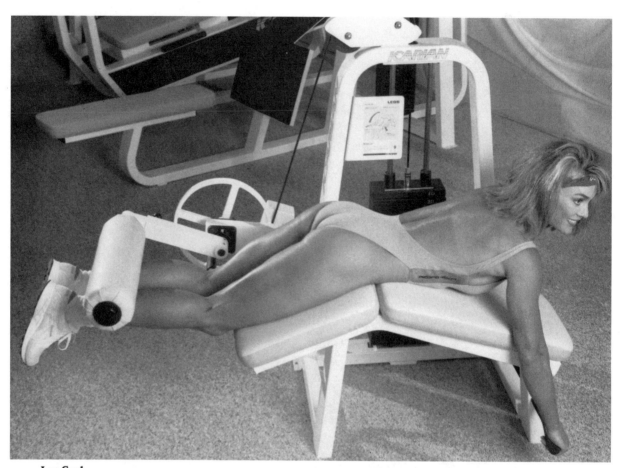

Leg Curl

B. Bend knees, pulling rollers toward buttocks and keeping hips on bench to avoid arching your back. Concentrate on the muscles you are working and visualize how shapely they will become.

C. Return to starting position and repeat.

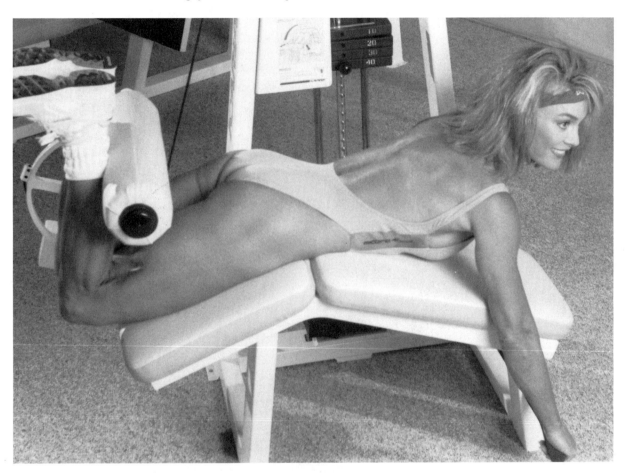

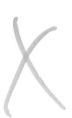

Leg extension and leg curls can also be done at home using ankle weights.

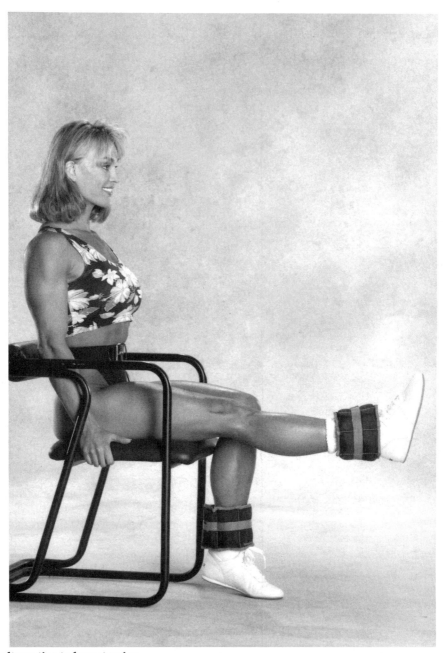

At-home alternative to leg extension.

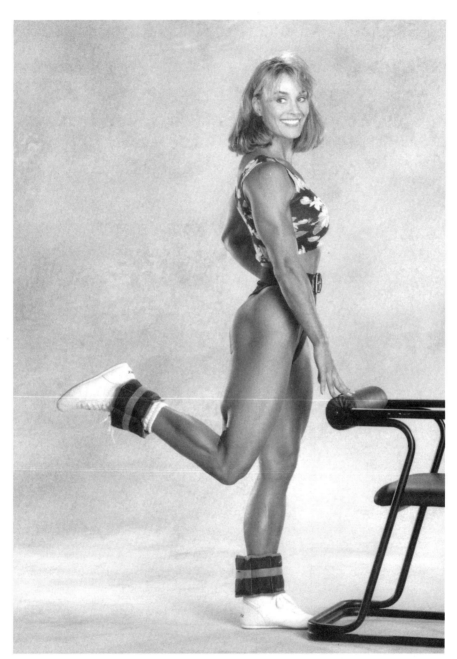

At-home alternative to leg curl.

4. LUNGES: Sculpts and strengthens many muscle groups in the quadriceps, glutes and upper hamstrings.

A. Take a comfortable step forward and slowly descend into a flexed knee position—the angle between your thigh and lower leg should not be more than 90 degrees.

B. Push back up to the starting position, stopping about 5–10 degrees short of a fully locked position.

*Tips: Do all reps on one leg before switching to the other for a more intense workout. Do without a barbell or weights if you're a beginner. Always concentrate on proper technique.

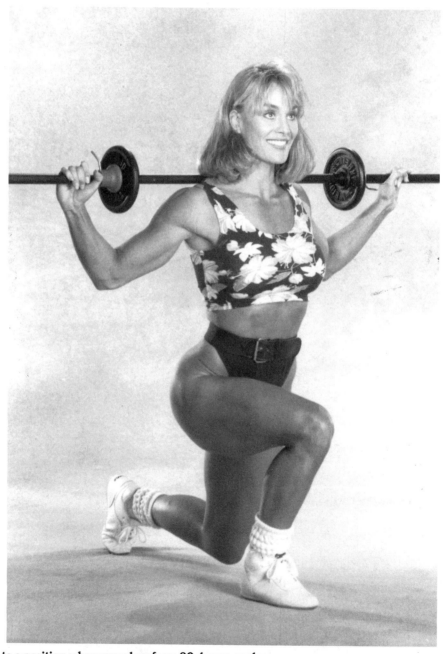

Go down to a position where your legs form 90 degree angles.

5. STANDING CALF RAISE: Sculpts and strengthens calves.

    A. Stand erect with one foot on a block of wood.
    B. Raise up on the ball of your foot board and hold for a second.
    C. Slowly lower yourself so that your heel goes well below the foot board.
    D. Alternate legs. Do all reps on one calf before you switch.

*Tips: Maximum height and depth is important for progress. Keep your knees just slightly bent when doing your raises. Work throughout a full range of motion and don't use so much weight that you strain your lower back. Breathe normally.

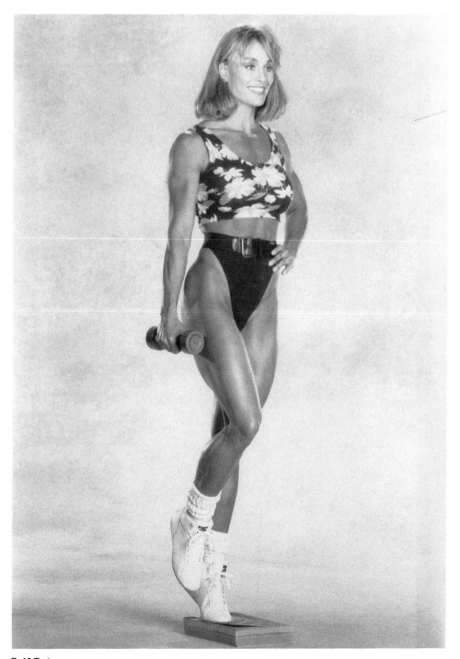

Standing Calf Raise

Two For a Beautiful, Strong Back

6. LAT PULL-DOWN: Sculpts and shapes and broadens your upper back or latissimus muscles.

 A. Start in a seated position facing the lat machine, with the tops of your thighs anchored under the upper seat.

 B. Grasp the overhead bar with a comfortable grip (slightly wider than shoulder width).

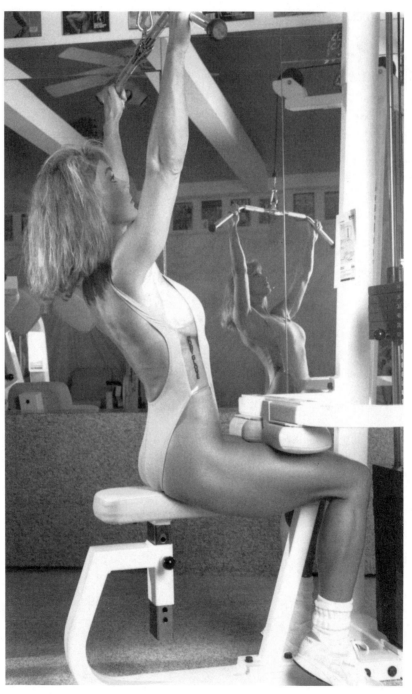

Lat Pull-down

C. Pull the bar down until it grazes the back of your neck/shoulder junction for behind the neck pull-downs, and to your upper chest for pull-downs to the front.

D. Keep your chest elevated and bring your elbows way back and down and think about squeezing your shoulder blades together.

*Tips: Pull-downs to the front are especially good for developing that sexy, broad back which will give the illusion of a smaller waist.

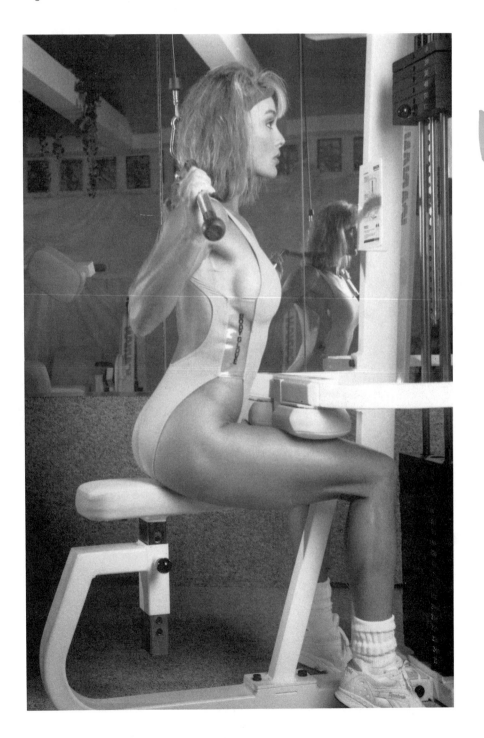

7. BENT-OVER ROW: Thickens out the muscles in the middle back.

   A. Bend over your barbell, keep your back just slightly higher than parallel to the ground, and maintain a 10–20 degree bend in your knees.

   B. Hold the bar with a pronated grip equal to your shoulder width and pull the bar up so that it touches your naval region.

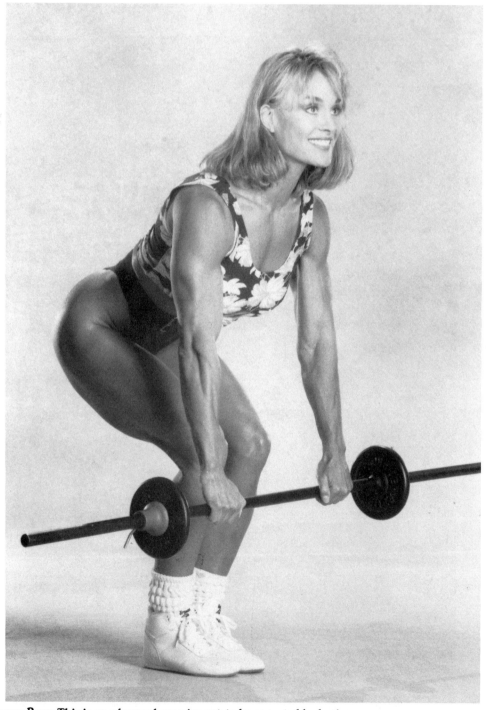

Bent-over Row: This is an advanced exercise not to be executed by beginners.

*Tips: Concentrate on keeping your back flat and draw your elbows way back and up. Don't yank the weight up or hold your breath.

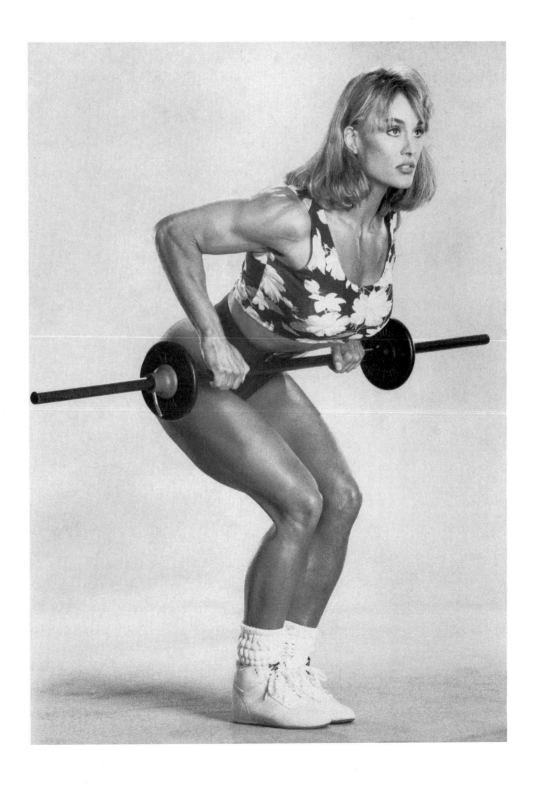

You can do a one-armed dumbbell row if you don't have barbells at home.

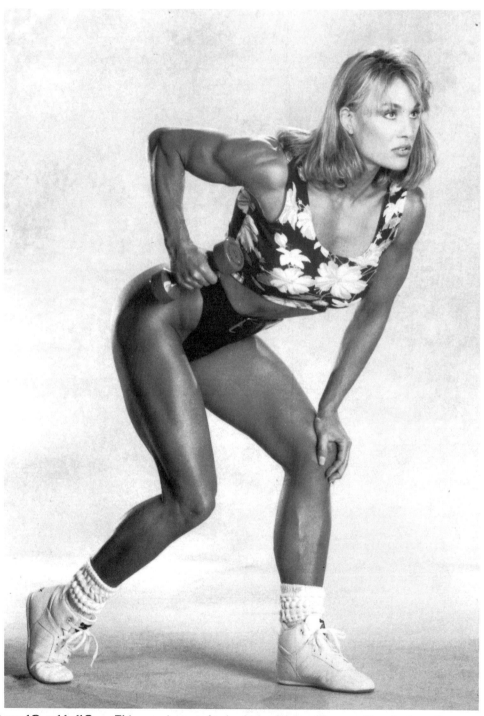

One-Armed Dumbbell Row: This exercise can also be done with your knee and hand supporting your weight on a bench.

Four for Beautiful Arms (Biceps and triceps)

8. SEATED CONCENTRATION CURL: Builds great biceps and is gentle on your back.

A. Sit on a flat bench holding a dumbbell with your extended arm bridged against the inside of your thigh.

B. Keeping your upper arm stationary, slowly curl the dumbbell up to your shoulder.

*Tips: Assist yourself with your opposite hand to squeeze out a few more reps.

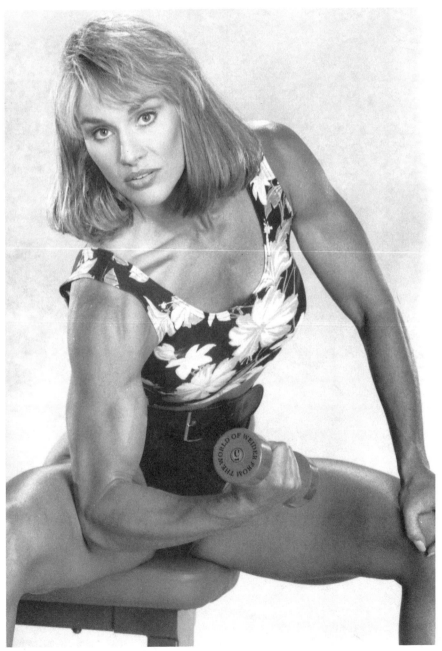

Seated Concentration Curl

9. DUMBBELL CURL: Also builds beautiful biceps.

    A. Sitting or standing, hold a dumbbell in each hand with your palms up.

    B. Slowly lift the dumbbells up, curling your lower arms up toward your shoulders.

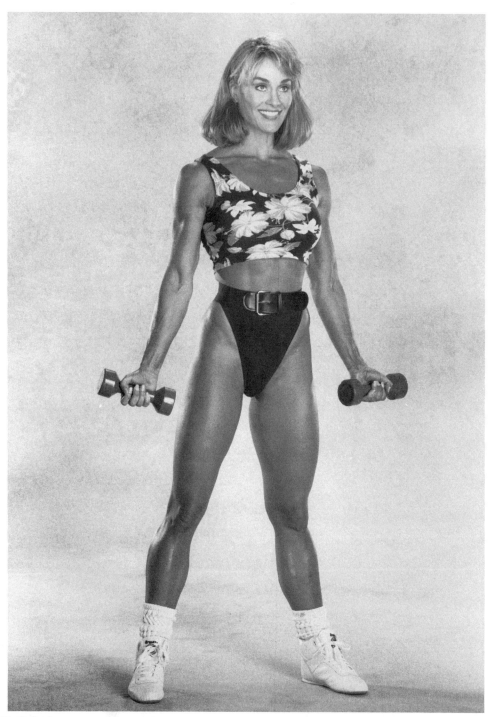

Dumbbell Curl

C. For another option, alternate arms, bring one dumbbell up, only after the other is all the way back down.

*Tips: Try to isolate only the bicep muscles. Do not swing the weight up–control it nice and slow.

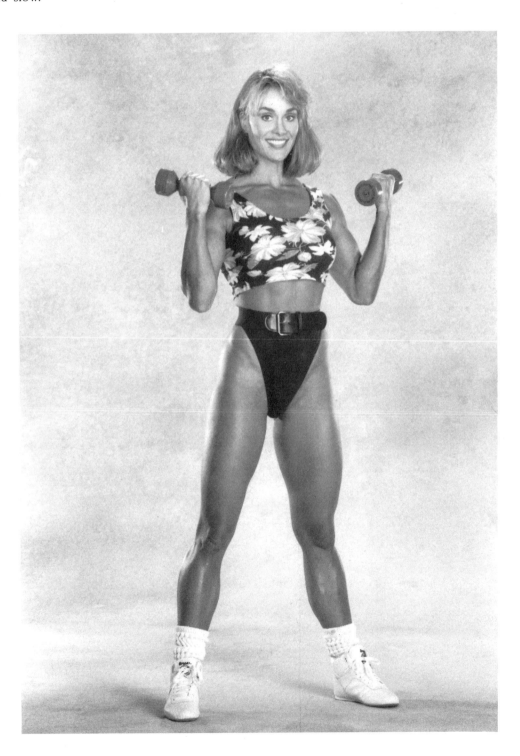

10. TRICEPS EXTENSIONS (SEATED): Works the belly of your three-headed triceps muscle (that muscle that gets flabby with age).

    A. While seated, position yourself on a bench holding a barbell and using a narrow, pronated grip.

    B. Push the bar up to arm's length.

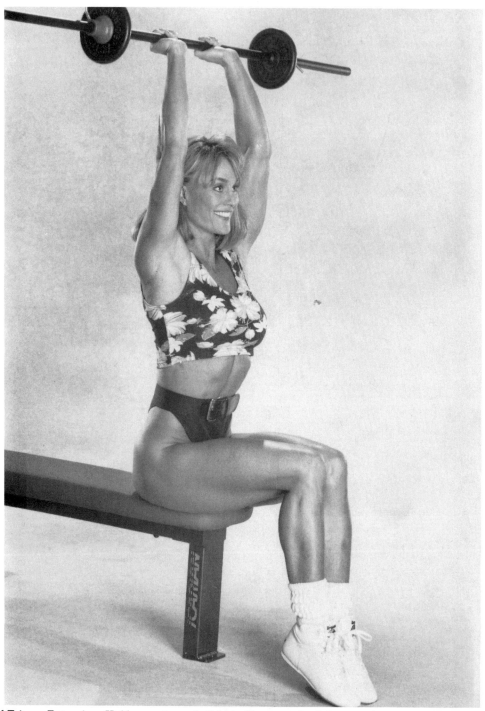

Seated Triceps Extension: Hold your stomach tight to keep your back from arching.

C. With your elbows stationary, lower the bar behind your head, keeping your upper arm stationary and close to your ears.

D. Straighten your elbows, returning the bar to the upright starting position.

*Tips: If seated, think about keeping your elbows fixed against your ears to isolate the triceps.

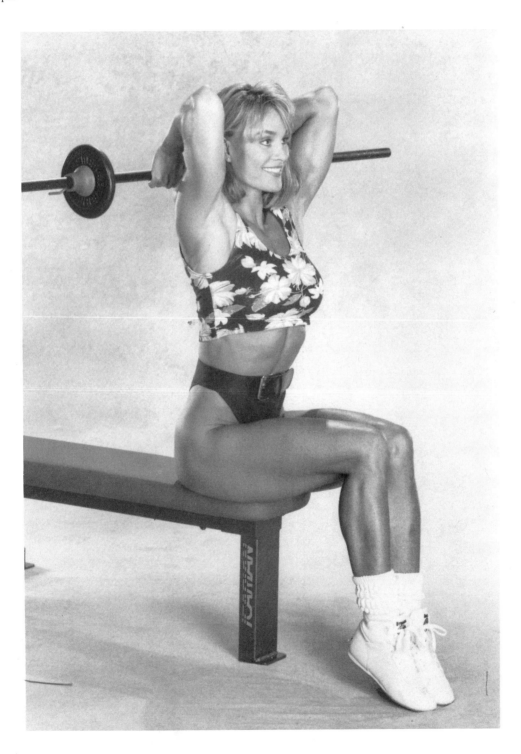

11. TRICEP KICKBACK: Works your triceps or muscles in the back of the arm.

A. Supporting yourself with one hand, kneel on a flat bench, hold a dumbbell with your other hand, and bend at your elbow.

B. Keeping your elbow fixed, move your lower arm back into extension until your arm is straight. Try not to move any part of your arm except your forearm.

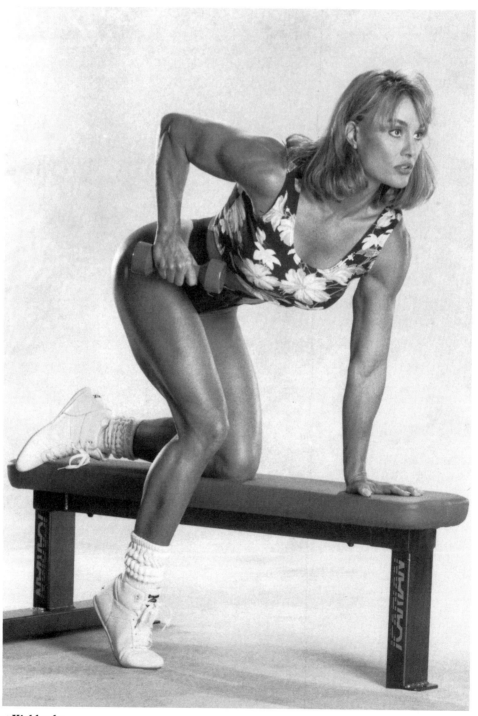

Triceps Kickbacks

C. Slowly lower the dumbbell back to the bent-elbow position. Do all reps on one arm before switching to the other.

*Tips: Especially good for firming up that part of the arm that keeps on waving long after you've said good-bye. Ladies, you don't need to use much weight here—higher repetitions and extremely strict form is the magic.

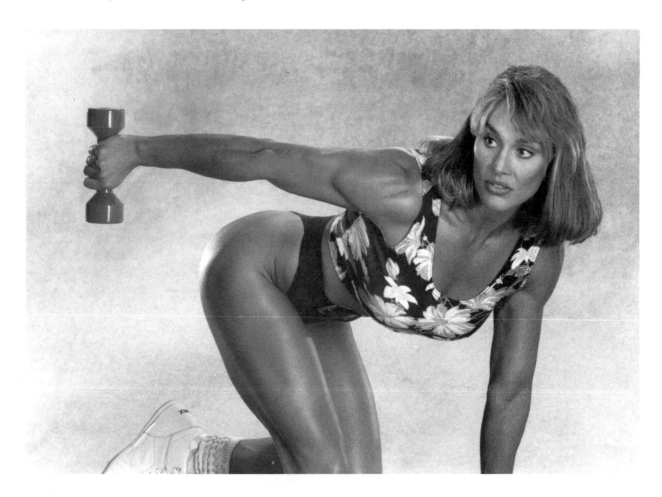

Two for Beautiful Shoulders

12. SEATED SHOULDER PRESS: Great for developing both shape and strength in the deltoids.

    A. Sit on bench with a dumbbell at each of your shoulders.
    B. Using a shoulder-width grip, press the dumbbells overhead to arm's length.

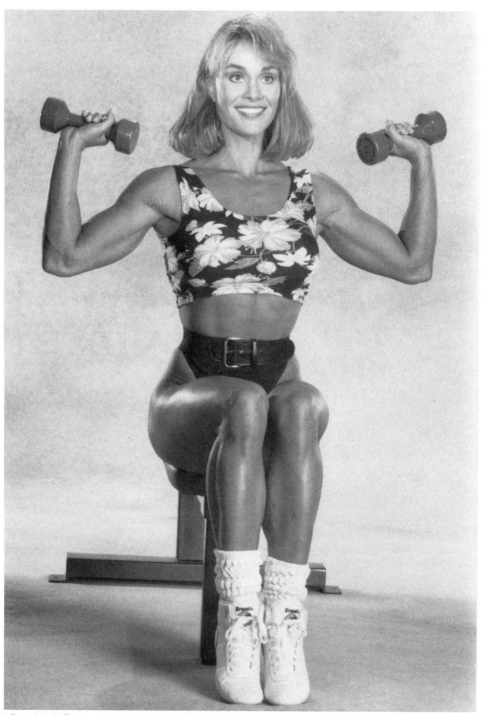

Seated Dumbbell Press

C. Breathe out as you press up and inhale as you slowly lower the bar back to your shoulders.

*Tips: As you press, plant your feet to maintain a solid body position. Keep your back straight, chest high.

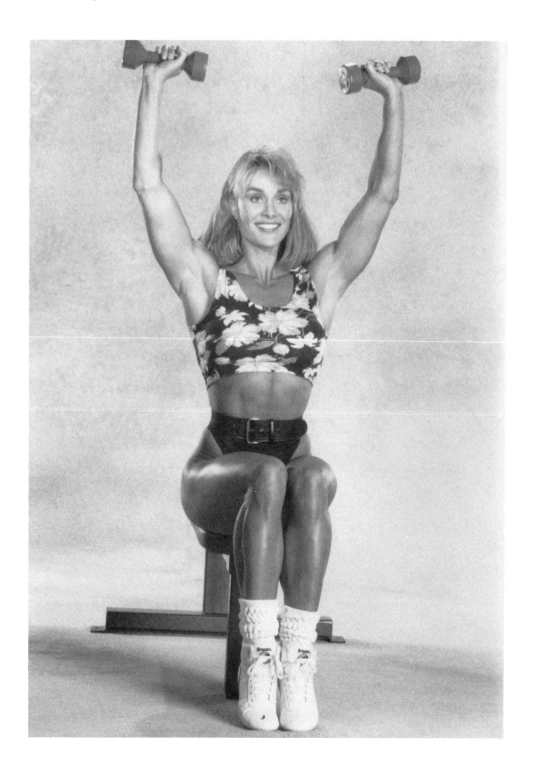

13. STANDING LATERAL RAISE (STANDING OR SITTING): For developing *width* to the shoulders.

A. Hold one dumbbell in each hand in front of your body, palms down, resting against your thighs.

B. Lean slightly forward and raise both dumbbells together to a level even with the top of your head.

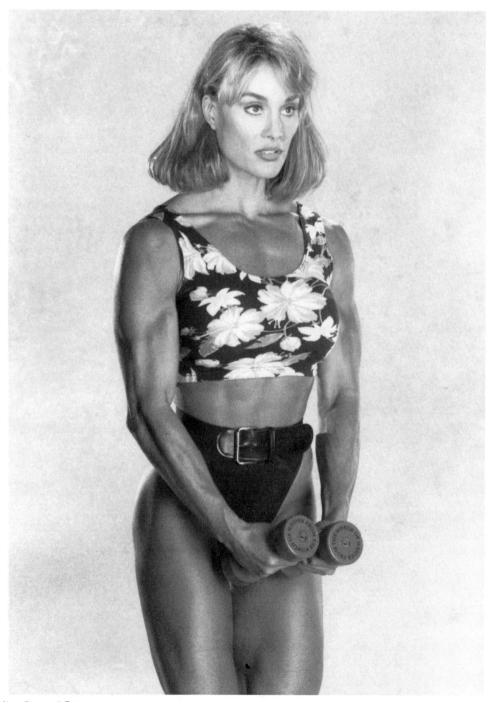

Standing Lateral Raise

C. As you raise the dumbbells, keep both elbows and wrist slightly flexed. Never let your wrist get higher than your elbows.

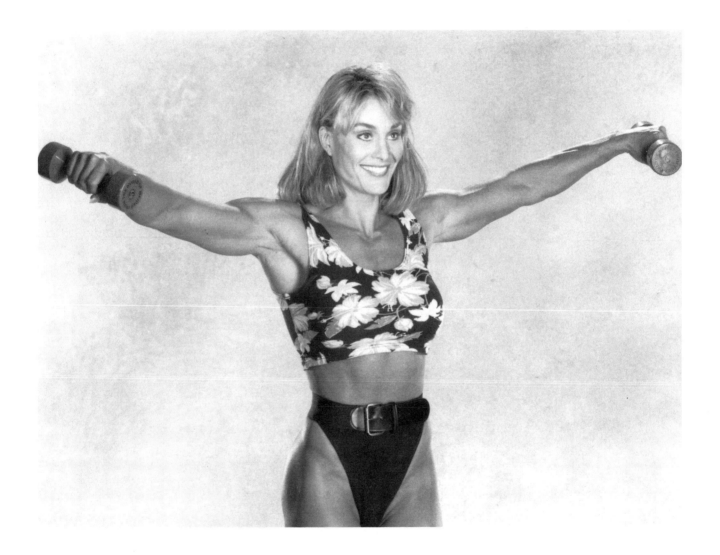

Two for Firm Abdominals

14. ABDOMINAL CRUNCH: Sculpts and strengthens front of torso.
     A. Lie on back with knees bent and feet up so thighs are perpendicular to floor. To support neck, cup your hands behind your head without intertwining fingers.

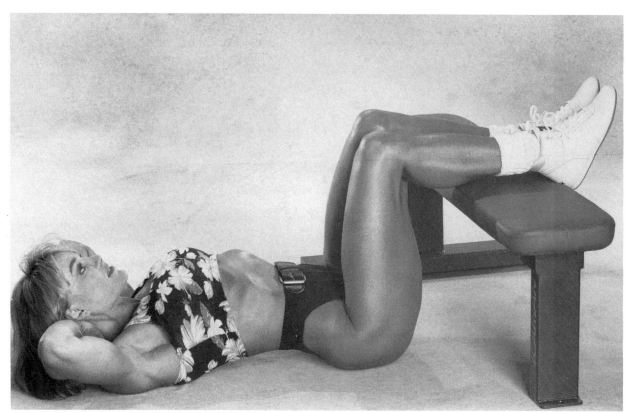

Abdominal Crunch

B. Lift head, neck, shoulders, and upper torso off the floor in one fluid motion until your shoulder blades clear the floor.

C. Exhale as you lift.

D. Return to starting position and repeat, maintaining your leg position.

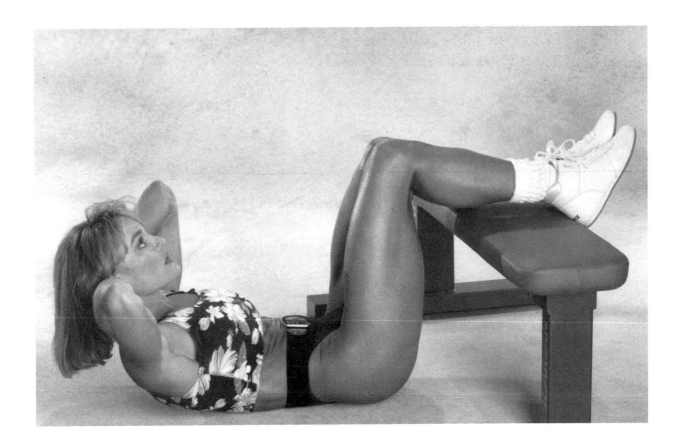

15. HYPEREXTENSIONS: This companion exercise strengthens your lower back to match your abdominal strength.

A. Lie face down on the floor, legs fully extended and arms by your side with your forehead resting comfortably on the floor.

B. Tighten buttocks muscles and tilt pelvis to pull tailbone down towards the floor.

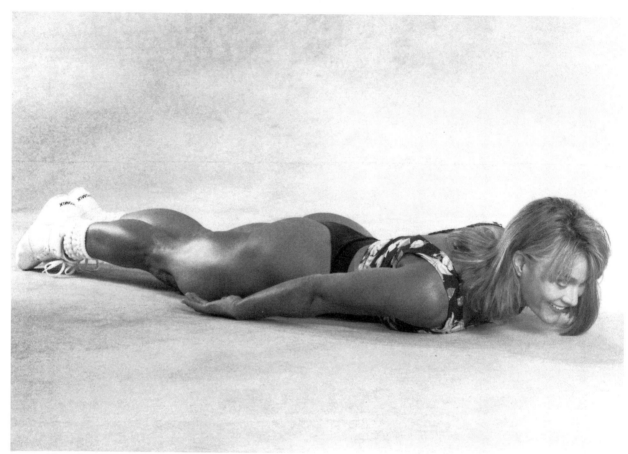

Floor Hyperextension: This is really good for firming your butt and lower back.

C. At the same time, lift upper torso 6 inches off floor, holding position for two counts. Return to starting position and repeat.

When you're ready, you can advance to a gym machine hyperextension. Also good for tightening up those sagging cheeks!

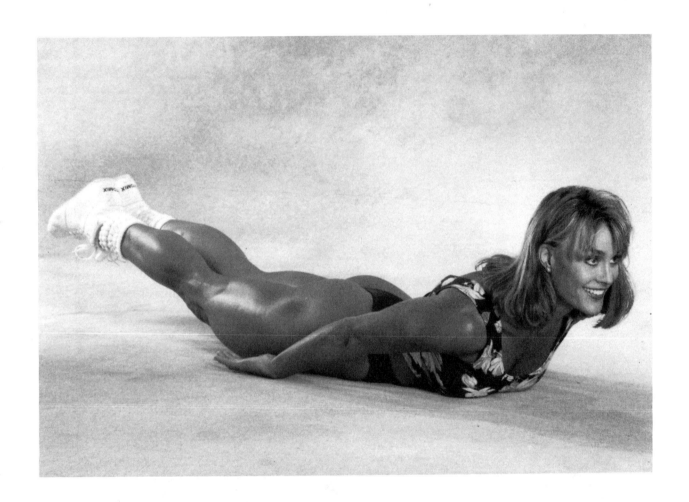

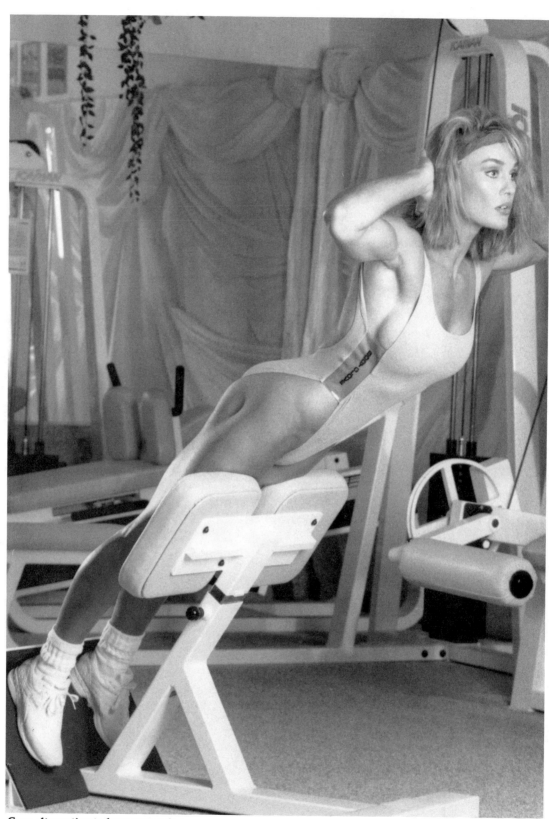

Gym alternative to hyperextension

Three to Build a More Shapely Chest

16. INCLINE DUMBBELL FLY

A. Lie on your back on the incline bench.

B. Press the dumbbells up to the top position, and hold them with your palms facing each other.

C. With a deep breath and keeping your chest held high, lower both dumbells to your sides through a wide arc while keeping your elbows slightly bent.

D. Lower the dumbbells to just below parallel with your body.

E. Exhale and bring the dumbbells back to the starting position along the same arc through which you lowered them. The movement should resemble a huge bear hug.

*Tips: You don't need much weight—do higher repetitions.

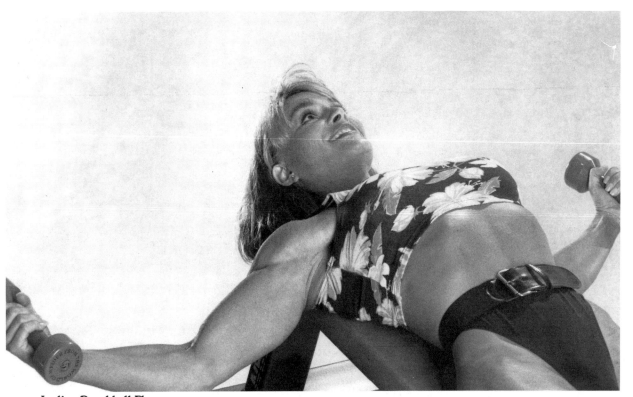

Incline Dumbbell Fly

17. INCLINE DUMBBELL PRESS: For the muscles in the upper chest or pectorals.

A. Position yourself on an incline bench that does not have supports, with two dumbbells at your feet, one on each side of the incline bench.

B. Bend down and lift the dumbbells up so that you are sitting on the incline bench with the dumbbells at your shoulders, ready to push up.

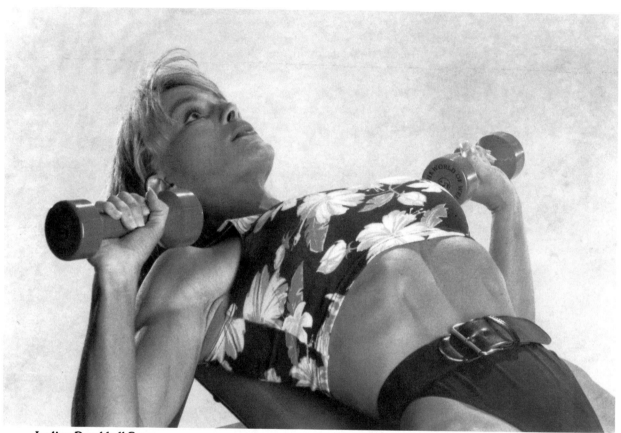

Incline Dumbbell Press

C. Push the dumbbells up together while breathing out. Keep your elbows out and your chest elevated so the emphasis is on your pectorals (chest muscles . . . remember Anatomy 101).

D. Inhale and lower the dumbbells together and press them up again. Go through a full range of motion.

*Tips: Never release the elevated chest position throughout your set. Lock into that position so only your arms are moving.

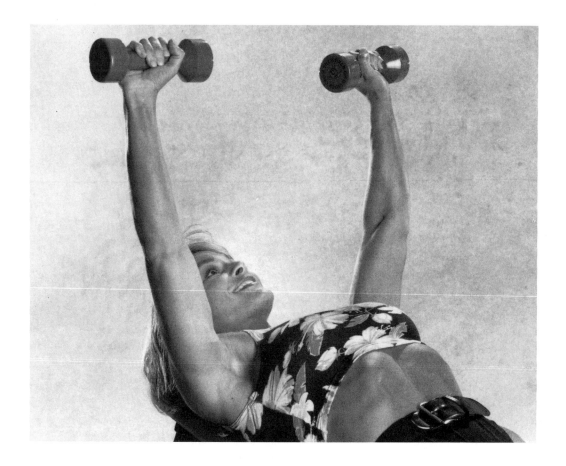

18. FLAT DUMBBELL PRESS: Strenghten those muscles and help stop the sagging process so you won't hang low or wobble to and fro!

    A. Lie on your back on a flat exercise bench.

    B. Pick up two dumbells and lie back on the bench with the dumbbells at chest/shoulder junction.

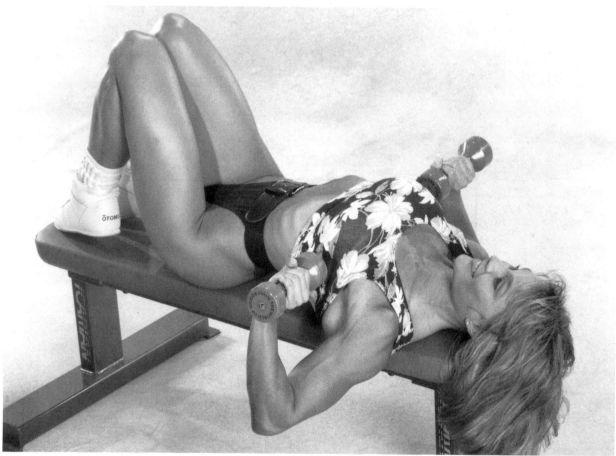

Flat Dumbbell Press

C. Push the dumbbells up together. Breathe out as you push them up and inhale as you lower them.

*Tips: Keep your elbows directed out to the sides perpendicular to the ground with a 90 degree angle at the elbow in the lowered position.

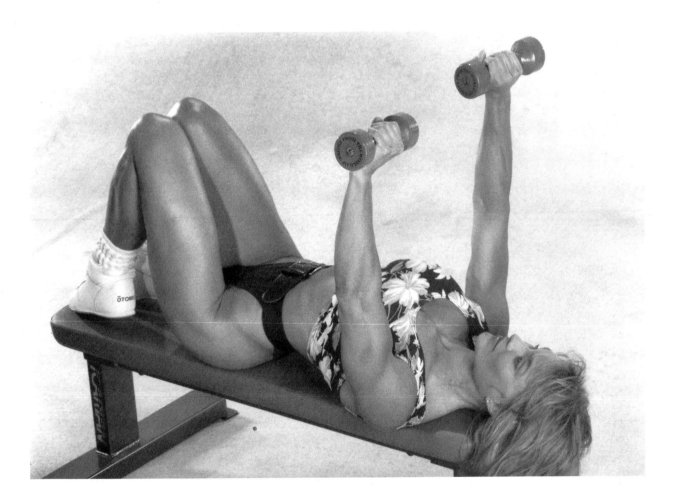

THE PROGRESSION GAME

How to move from beginner to intermediate to advanced? Easy! You simply use the same exercises I used to become Ms. Olympia six times straight. The only difference between my workout and yours is the number of sets and amount of weight you'll use.

Beginners

One to two sets of each exercise, with 10–20 reps for lower body exercises and 10–15 reps for upper body. Rest 35 to 40 seconds between sets. When you can do two sets of 12 reps comfortably, add a third, increasing to 15 reps per set over a period of two to four weeks. When this is comfortable, increase weight by 5–10 pounds and decrease reps to 10, progressing back up to 15 reps for each set. Allow about three weeks for this progression. When you can easily do three sets of 15 reps at the new weight, progress to intermediate.

*Beginner Tips: Learn to concentrate on form and technique and feel the muscle working in the specific muscle group you are training. Be patient. The lower body can handle more reps than the upper body because it has larger, stronger muscle groups. Did you know the butt muscle (gluteus) is the largest muscle in the body—quite obvious on some of us.

Intermediates

Do two to three sets, per body part, of 10 to 12 reps, resting 30 to 45 seconds between sets. Gradually increase the reps to 15 per set. When this is comfortable, increase weight by 5–10 pounds and reduce reps back to 10, progressing back up to 15. Repeat progression of increasing weight and decreasing reps and working back up to 15 reps. Allow four to six weeks to progress. When you can easily do four sets of 15, move up to advanced.

Advanced

Do three to five sets, per body part, with more weight, with 10–20 reps for lower body and 10–15 reps for your upper body. If you can't use more weight, maintain perfect technique, then simply do more repetitions, which also increases your training intensity.

Remember, move smoothly and quickly from exercise to exercise. Don't blab in the gym about your weekend happenings—get your workout done first! The less rest you take, the more aerobic your workout will be and the quicker you get out of the gym and on with your day. Don't waste time! Be efficient so your day won't be deficient. Besides, who wants to spend all day in the gym?

And remember: K.I.S.S.: Keep It Simple, Sweetheart. Stick to the basics—I always did and enjoyed consistent success. Don't listen to goofballs who swear by fancy moves.

CORY'S THREE-DAY TOTAL-BODY SCULPTING AND STRENGTH-BUILDING WORKOUT (30 MINUTES A DAY, 60–90 MINUTES A WEEK)

In this workout, you train your entire body every time you workout. Do it three days a week, with aerobics and rest days in between so your muscles can recoup. It burns fat (if you move from set to set without breaks), tones muscles, and sculpts a more beautiful body. So what are you waiting for?

Stretch and warm up (see Chapter 7)

1. Squats or lunges: 1–3 sets; 10–20 reps
2. Leg Extensions: same
3. Leg curls: same
4. One Arm Dumbbell Row; 1–3, 10–15 sets
   (add pull-downs if at gym)
5. Incline Dumbbell Press: same
6. Flat Bench Fly: same
7. Behind the Neck Press: 1–3 sets, 8–15 reps
8. Lateral Raise: same
9. Dumbbell Curl or Concentration Curl: 1–3 sets; 10–15 reps
10. Tricep Extensions or Kickback: same
11. Abdominal Crunches: 1–3 sets; 25–50 reps
12. Hyperextensions: 1–3 sets; 10–20 reps
    (Alternate one set crunches with one set hyperextensions.)

CORY'S THREE-DAY SPLIT BODY SCULPTING AND STRENGTHENING WORKOUT

In this workout, you train different body parts on three alternating days, focusing on upper body one day a week and lower body two days a week.

Day One: chest, shoulders, triceps, and abdominals

Day Two: Thighs, hamstrings, butt, and lower back

Day Three: Back, biceps, and abdominals. On the other days, do 20–30 minutes of aerobic exercise.

DAY ONE:

Stretch and warm up
1. Bench Press; 2–4 sets; 10–15 reps
2. Incline Press: same
3. Flys: same
4. Behind the Neck Press; 2–4 sets; 8–15 reps
5. Lateral Raises: same
6. Tricep Extensions (or pushdowns if at gym) 2–4 sets; 10–15 reps
7. Tricep Kickback: same
8. Abdominal Crunches: 2–4; 50 reps

DAY TWO

Stretch and warm up
1. Squat: 2–5 sets; 10–20 reps
2. Leg Extensions: same
3. Leg Curl: same
4. Lunges: same
5. Hyperextensions (can add 5 pounds behind head if desired): same
6. Calves: same
7. Abdominals: 2–4 sets; 20–50 reps

DAY THREE

Stretch and warm up
1. One-arm Bent-over Row: 2–5 sets; 10–15 reps
2. Lat Pull-downs if at gym or chin-ups if at home: same
3. Long Pulley Row if at gym: same
4. Flatback Deadlifts with dumbbells: same
5. Alternate Dumbbell Curls: same
6. Seated Concentration Curls: same
7. Abdominal Crunches: 2–4 sets; 20–50 reps
8. Hyperextensions: 2–4 sets; 1–20 reps
   (Alternate one set crunches with one set hyperextensions.)

RX FOR INJURY PREVENTION

If you are careful and train smart, you will not hurt yourself during training. Most injuries are as minor as a slight muscle pull, if that. But neglect and delay can turn a minor injury into a major one.

Even small injuries warrant medical attention. Unless your name ends in "M.D.", this is no time to play Mrs. Fix-It.

- Keep fingers and toes away from moving parts of machines.
- Always make sure the collars are tightly fastened on free weights.
- If you suddenly feel weak but have no pain, or if you experience unusual swelling or bruising, see the doctor.
- Never "work through" an injury. Stop exercising immediately.
- Elevate the injured area to minimize swelling and internal bleeding.
- Apply ice right away to help decrease swelling and bleeding, but not right on your skin—ice can burn, too. Wrap the ice in a thin towel.
- If the injury was accompanied by audible popping or tearing, don't move or put weight on the injured part and see a doctor right away.
- Ask your physician about taking aspirin to relieve inflammation.
- Follow your doctor's instruction for rest and supplemental treatment, e.g., ultrasound, massage, or physical therapy.

- Don't go back to training until you're completely healed. Before your workout, take a long, hot shower to relax your muscles, do some light stretches, and then work out using slow, careful motions with light weights. Do lots of reps with a full range of motion to encourage blood flow to the area to aid healing.

Once an area is injured, it's more vulnerable to subsequent injuries. If possible, avoid the exercise which resulted in the injury and substitute something that puts less strain on the muscle.

BUILDING YOUR OWN HOME GYM

After waiting an hour last week to use the Nautilus machines—and another half hour for your turn on the stair climber, you've decided enough is enough. It's time for a home gym.

Beware: It's a gym jungle out there in exercise-machine land, with a con on every corner. Which machines to buy? Here are a few suggestions for aerobic and weight-training machines that won't leave you stranded or stuck with a broken-down machine that winds up as a high-priced clothes hanger.

GREAT SWEATS

Okay, first things first. What's your aerobic motion of choice? If it's running or walking, try a stair climber or treadmill. For a great total-body workout, nothing beats a rowing or cross-country machine. Or if you prefer to ride your calories away, a stationary bike or even a recumbent stationary bike that you pedal with your legs stretched out in front of you is your best bet since it puts less strain on your lower back.

However you decide to move it, your first step is a serious fitness dealer. Forget fly-by-nighters. Before taking it home, give the machine a test drive, just as you would a new car. (Some of these machines cost almost as much!)

Here are a few general rules to follow when buying machines.

NUTS AND BOLTS OF GREAT MACHINES

- Avoid machines with lots of play or slack in the movement.
- Make sure you can easily make adjustments or change from one exercise to the next.
- Don't be wowed by fancy gadgets and computers. Sometimes the best machines are the simplest—and if you're a beginner, those bells and whistles are likely to intimidate, confuse, and most of all, distract.
- Ride/pedal/row or whatever for at least 10 minutes to make sure it's comfortable and doesn't have any bad moves or kinks.
- You get what you pay for: Don't expect a $200 does-everything "deal" to deliver a good workout. It probably will be a bumpy, clunky gadget that breaks down because you tossed it into the wall out of frustration.
- How to spot a loser: Ever notice how many of those machines you see at garage sales seem to be the same name brands? Avoid them like the plague.

- Look for machines that offer a good stretch and full extension. (See definitions on p. 177)
- Don't let a salesperson con or power talk you. They're paid to sell, period. Try out the machines first for a good feel and choose the one you like. Everyone has slightly different limb lengths, so what fits the salesperson may not necessarily fit you.

WORKOUT TIPS FOR HOME-ALONERS

1. With no one watching, you may be tempted to put off your home-exercise program. If you want the machine to work for you, you have to use it. Set up a schedule and stick to it.

2. Be real. Set attainable goals and go for them. Don't expect to be Ms. Olympia on an hour a week.

3. Give yourself a break. (Not literally speaking, of course.) What we mean is, don't give up if you don't see immediate results. Allow at least a month for those pretty little biceps to begin to pop out or for your bottom line to show signs of recession. Don't be overzealous or you'll find yourself poring over our Rx for Injury Prevention section on page 220.

4. Of course you have time. We're talking less than four hours a week here, girls—20 to 30 minutes, three days a week—or less time than some of us spend each day on our hair. You want your body to look as good? You know what to do.

5. While we're on the subject of poor excuses, forget the tight budget bit, too. All you need for any of these workouts is a set of free weights (about $10) and a kitchen bench (if you don't have one, try Goodwill or the Salvation Army; $5 tops). As for the rest of the exercises—pushups, situps, crunches, they're free.

6. Keep your machine up and out if possible. You know the old saying: Out of sight out of mind. And when it comes to exercise equipment—out of shape.

Enough on exercise and nutrition. One last chapter to wrap things up and you're ready to go!

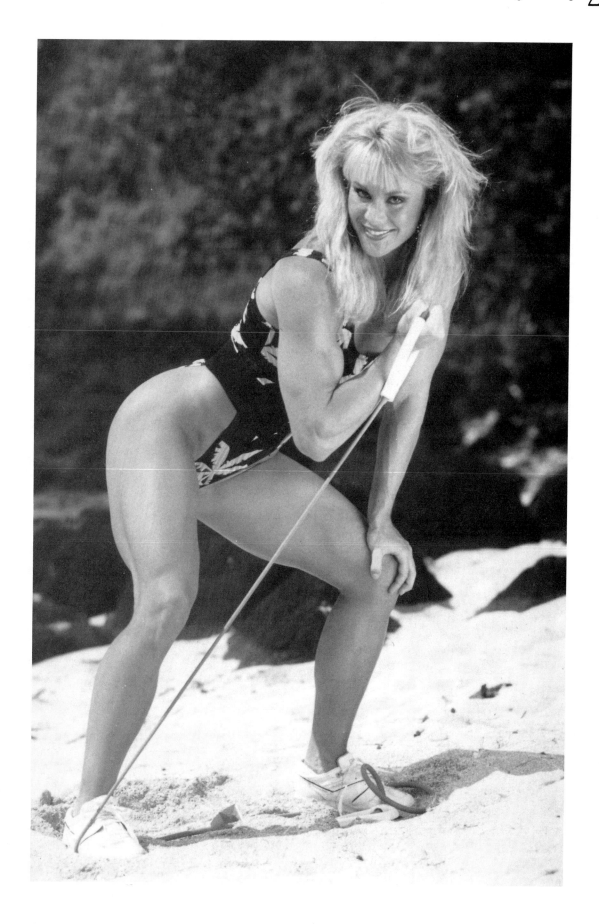

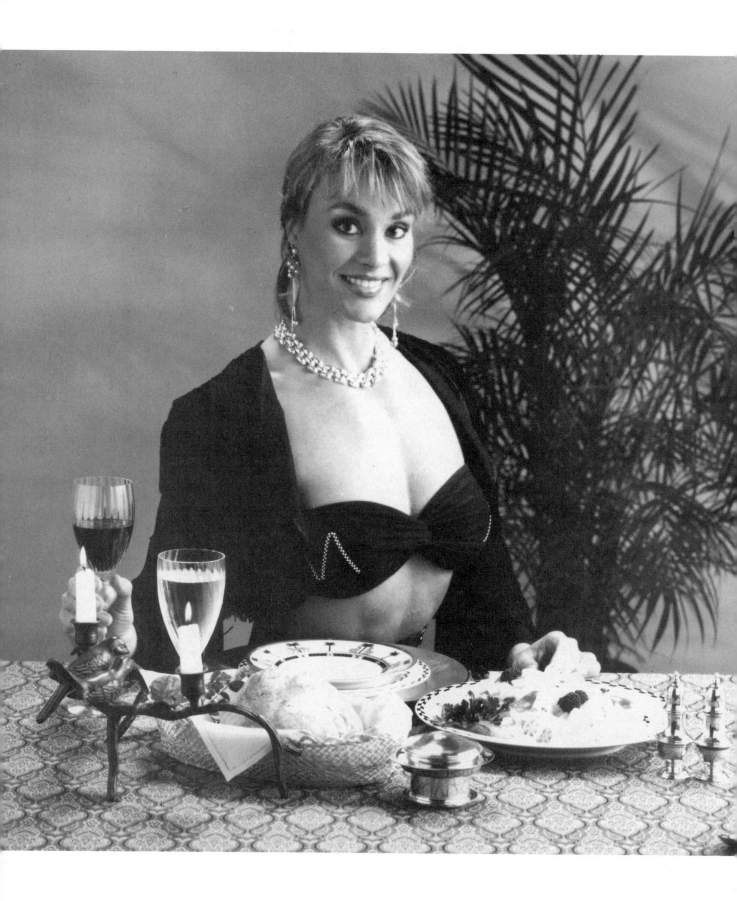

Ten

Low-Fat Survival in a High-Fat World

What's a girl gotta do to maintain a firm tush in a world where fat oozes from every flat surface? Wear blinders and nose plugs? Avoid all streets with bakeries and pizzerias?

Whether your challenge is shunning the cheesecake at the holiday ball or reuniting with your waistline après pregnancy, this chapter can give you the low-fat tips you need to keep your newly-slim physique in a world that often seems like a perverse conspiracy to plump it back out. Let's start with eating out. Careful, ladies: It's a junk food jungle out there.

DINE OUT WITHOUT DOING YOURSELF IN

Read between the menu lines at your favorite family restaurant and you'll find that many otherwise low-fat foods are pushed overboard into the high-calorie danger zone by the way they're prepared.

A virgin baked potato is a low-fat feast at 150 calories and zero fat. Unfortunately, it's often served swimming in butter and sour cream (as if just one wasn't bad enough). Watch out for "stuffed vegetables," too; if they're stuffed with stuffing, you're back to square one.

And what could be more low-fat and healthful than fish? Seems like a conspiracy. By the time the grinning waiter gets it to your table, it's so heavily breaded and deep-fried that the fish seems like an afterthought–you might as well be eating French fries.

In fact, a typical restaurant meal consisting of fried mushrooms, a 10-ounce steak, large baked potato with sour cream, plus buttered peas and cheesecake contains about 2,000 calories–more than many women's daily caloric intake, and more than enough fat for an entire week!

Substitute a salad for the fried mushrooms, broiled chicken for steak, steamed vegetables for buttered corn, and a slice of angel food for the cheesecake, and you've cut the damage by more than 1,200 calories—or the number of calories in breakfast and lunch—and nearly eliminated the larger evil: fat.

LOW-FAT BUZZWORDS

When you open a menu, look for the low-fat buzzwords that signal that food has been prepared without added fat. These include such words as broiled, steamed, poached, garden-fresh, cooked in its own juice, tomato sauce, roasted, marinated in juice or wine, charbroiled, boiled, barbecued, stir-fried, mesquite-grilled.

If it's fried, crispy, buttery, creamed, in its own gravy, cream sauce, au gratin, in cheese sauce or stuffed with cheese, marinated in oil or butter, served "Scampi" style, breaded, stuffed or served with meat or cheese sauce, sautéed, Alfredo, and pan-fried, you can bet it's swimming in fat. Steer clear, or at least tread lightly.

THE CUSTOMER IS ALWAYS RIGHT

Don't be shy. Ask the chef to prepare food your way. As a paying customer, it's your right, and most chefs will be delighted to do it for you. You might want to call in advance, just to make sure that the chef has the time to accommodate your order.

ORDERING THE LOW-FAT WAY

Of course there are times it's impossible to order the low-fat way. Some diners deserved to be called "greasy spoon" because the cook prepares food only one way, his way. But low-life eateries aren't the only high-fat culprits. Many a hoity-toity Chez à la Grease charges big bucks for a plateful of fat. Both ends of the dining spectrum call for creative ordering and close scrutiny of the menu at hand.

Even greasy-spoon joints usually have some low-fat items amid the fried, breaded, and creamed offerings. If not, cut corners where possible.

KEEPING DOWN THE FAT TAB

Gayle Shockey Hoxter has turned eating in the "fat lane" into a fine science. Here are a few of the tricks she uses to maintain her trim figure.

- When dining out, forget what Mother once said about cleaning your plate. Most restaurants serve enough food for you and Mom.
- Scout out restaurants with lower-fat menus and try to avoid grease pits. Hint: you can usually smell them a mile away.
- The all-you-can-eat buffet is the bane of dieters, so don't be greedy just because you can eat as much as you want "for free." You know the old saying—there's no such thing as a "fat-free" lunch. You pay for it in the end, which is where it usually sticks.

- If you're going to be on the road for a while, stash a diner's survival kit in your glove box: artificial sweeteners, packets of low-fat dressing, mustard, Butter Buds or Molly McButter, Mrs. Dash, herbs, and even a greasy spoon diner meal can be transformed into low-fat eating.
- Tell the waiter to bring bread with the meal; otherwise you may do as I do and eat a loaf or two before the meal even arrives.

TWENTY LOW-FAT SURVIVAL TIPS

We asked several food experts to share their favorite eating/cooking secrets with you.

1. Make Every Bite Count

How fast you eat can be as important as what you eat when it comes to reducing the amount of high-fat foods in your diet. Studies show that the human brain requires 20 minutes to register satiety, no matter what or how much you eat. That means the slower you eat, the less food you require to feel full. Fill up first on foods that take time to sip or chew and you'll not only be pleasantly full but less likely to overindulge on more fattening subsequent courses.

2. Weigh the Damage

Whether that chicken breast weighs three ounces or four is something that only your food scale knows for sure. Invest in a scale and you could help prevent unmeasured ounces from turning into unwanted pounds. Use it for a month or two until you get into the smaller-portion habit.

3. A Taste'll Do Ya

Debbie Fields, baker of those famously addictive cookies, is one smart cookie. Instead of letting the chips weigh her down (not to mention the butter), she takes a nibble or two and that's it. Try it and a bite or two will keep the cookie monster (or whatever high-fat fiend you're battling) at bay.

4. Avoid Midnight Snack Attacks

Studies show that late-hour calories tend to hang around longer than those you consume earlier in the day because you don't have a chance to work them off through exercise. If you're a night owl, unless you sleepwalk or work the night shift, don't eat too much after about 8 P.M.

5. Don't Skip Breakfast

Too busy to grab a bite for breakfast? This is the age of the commuter mug, remember? Whirl a smoothie together, grab a bagel, and hi-ho. You know the alternatives.

6. Think Before You Bite

How quickly we forget about the chips and dip we wolf down in front of the tube, or the buttered popcorn we crunch at the movies. Unfortunately, your body never forgets. In fact, you might as well sit in fat because that's where it sticks. Bring Popcorn Rice Cakes to the movies like I do.

7. Veg Out

Remove meat and dairy products from your diet, and you automatically cut 90 percent of the fat. Don't go cold turkey; it could trigger a binge. Instead, try a gradual transition from meat to a vegan diet that allows your body and taste buds to adjust to new tastes, textures and less fat.

8. Brush Your Teeth or Gargle

If the urge to snack attacks, before you reach the kitchen, brush your teeth or gargle. It'll temporarily postpone the craving, and who wants to ruin a fresh, clean mouth with more food?

9. Keep a Food Diary

You'll be amazed at what you eat, and a diary can point up helpful patterns; for instance, nervous or moody eating. Also, knowing that you'll have a permanent record around will likely make you think before you chew. (Hide the white out, ladies!)

10. Sabotage Cravings

You're absolutely dying for a piece of cake. If you don't have one right now, you'll . . . die? I don't think so. Try taking a brisk jog—aerobic exercise has a way of dulling your appetite (especially if you don't really have one to begin with).

11. Don't Skip Meals

Eat something every three hours: a rice cake, a piece of fruit, anything healthful to take the edge off your appetite.

12. Eat Up to Six Times As Much Carbohydrates As Protein

Stock up on rice, pasta, baked potatoes, vegetables, fruits, breads, and grains. Eat at least five times more of these than protein foods such as fatty meats and whole-fat dairy products. Most of us get enough protein, and the excess doesn't turn it into muscle but fat.

13. Forget the 30-Percent Rule

If you'd like to eat a piece of chocolate cake that contains 45 percent calories from fat, enjoy it. Just cut back on fat the next day. That way, you can have your cake and still adhere to the 30-percent fat rule for the week.

14. Be a Muncher

A few potato chips or cookies here and there can creep up on you, even if you eat sensibly at mealtime, so stock your refrigerator and cupboards with munchies that contain no more than 50 to 70 calories per serving: air-popped popcorn, melba toast with low-calorie jam, fresh-fruit, vegetables, sugar-free hot chocolate, or sugar-free soda. Or make party snacks (even if it's only a party for you!), such as frozen pineapple chunks on toothpicks, fruit kabobs, or non-fat cream cheese on celery.

15. Feed the Right Hunger

Ask yourself this question the next time you reach for another cookie. Am I really hungry?

Many people eat for reasons that have nothing to do with physical hunger, according to John Foreyt, Ph.D., director of the Nutrition Research Clinic at the Baylor School of Medicine in Houston and the author of *Living Without Dieting* (Houston: Harrison Publishing, 1992).

Depression, anxiety, elation, even boredom can trigger a raid on the refrigerator. Unfortunately, most foods eaten to satisfy emotional hunger are high in fat. To distinguish one hunger from another, eat five or six healthful mini meals daily. That way, you'll never give your body a chance to feel true hunger. If you're still snacking, you're probably feeding the wrong hunger.

16. RX for Travel

Sometimes unexpected food situations arise without warning. Tuck a few low-fat energy bars into your purse, some low-fat cheese and crackers, perhaps some carrot and celery sticks and you're ready to fly the fattening skies.

17. Never Shop Hungry

You're likely to load the cart with junk food and snack on it all the way to the check-out counter.

18. Never Party Hungry

Who knows when dinner will be served—it could be midnight. Eat a high-carbohydrate snack before leaving home and you'll be less likely to overdose on hors d'oeuvres or overeat when dinner is served.

19. Avoid Calories on High:

A typical airline meal packs 1,200 calories and mucho fat. Call ahead and order a special or vegetarian meal and make low-fat snacks a standard part of your carry-on luggage.

20. When in Rome . . .

Here's a brief sampler of what to eat/not eat in ethnic restaurants:

American: Choose items noted by a heart, which means they meet standards set by the American Heart Association.

Mexican: Avoid taco salads, beef tacos and burritos, enchiladas, refried beans, and anything with guacamole—mucho fat! Instead, order marinated seafood, regular cooked beans, chicken burritos with salsa, and baked corn tortillas.

Chinese: Use your noodle and avoid duck, fried noodles, egg rolls, and anything breaded and fried—for instance fried shrimp. Try stir-fried vegetables, steamed rice dishes, and broiled fish.

Italian: Order pasta with a little tomato sauce, minestrone soup, anything in a marinara sauce, such as fish, Italian ice for dessert. Avoid stuffed pasta shells, ravioli, lasagna, and garlic bread or aie mama! You could become a regular meatball.

Indian: Low in protein and high in carbohydrates and fiber, Indian fare can be a godsend provided you avoid the ghee (clarified butter), fritters, and creamy curry sauce. Try Tandoori chicken and fish, lentil dishes, and pulkas (breads).

French: This country's rich sauces, croissants, and desserts can be Doomsday to your diet. Order simple dishes without the rich sauces and fill up on French bread, which is low in fat.

HOLIDAY SURVIVAL GUIDE

Uh oh. Here comes Santa Claus, and if we're not careful over the holidays, we'll wind up looking like *him*.

The holidays don't have to be a calorie nightmare. Arm yourself with our holiday survival guide and you'll be able to say ho! ho! ho! to holiday temptations without running away to the North Pole to chill 'til the party's over. Here are twelve easy ways.

THE TWELVE DAYS OF YOUR SURVIVAL GUIDE

1. Easy on the booze. The caloric damage from alcohol lingers long after the hangover lifts; new studies show calories from alcohol are the most difficult to burn. Also, that alcohol enhances your body's tendency to store fat.

2. You know that 10-ton fruitcake you've always eaten just because it's festive—even though you hate it? This year stockpile your "treat calories" for things you really enjoy: a piece of fudge, a few butter cookies, a glass of champagne.

3. Company for dinner? Don't pick-pick-pick as you cook and stir. Chew a wad of gum to keep your mouth preoccupied, send guests home with doggy bags (Rover never had it so good), or stash leftovers you can't give away in meal-sized doggy bags for quick meals that go from freezer to microwave in a flash.

4. So many friends, too many calories? Chow down too many holiday dinners and you'll wind up looking like a stuffed turkey yourself. Rather than eating an entire meal at any one sitting, eat a series of mini-meals, loading your plate with the least fattening items (fresh vegetables, fruit, white (not dark) meat, and mashed potatoes without gravy and butter.

5. Don't let your exercise program cramp your holiday spirit—or schedule. Instead of cramming your regular workout into a hectic holiday schedule, be flexible and go with the festive flow: Take a brisk hike, engage in some fast-paced aerobic window-shopping, or take up

a new winter sport, such as ice skating, cross-country skiing, or sledding. Finally, lower your expectations a little during the holidays. No one's counting how many cookies you eat. Remember: It takes an extra 3,500 calories to gain one pound. That's 35 cookies—or a whole box at once.

EXPECTING SOMEONE?

You're pregnant. How to eat for two? In a word—don't.

In fact, most women of average weight don't need to consume more than an extra 300 calories a day during pregnancy—that's a banana, two slices of toast with a teaspoon of peanut butter, and a glass of skim milk.

Overeating will only make you fatter—and could lead to problems during pregnancy and delivery. Starve yourself, however, and you could also starve your baby with disastrous results. A lack of protein and calories in the last trimester can interfere with brain development while too little folic acid has been linked to spinal defects. Fasting late in pregnancy may trigger premature birth.

If you suffer from or are recuperating from an eating disorder, including anorexia, bulimia, or laxative abuse, tell your doctor so he can help you correct deficiencies before they hurt your baby.

IS IT SAFE TO EXERCISE?

In the old days, the doctor put you to bed when you became pregnant—or at least told you to "take it easy." No more! Today, athletes and very fit women often exercise up to the day of delivery, although most taper off during the third trimester, limiting workouts to stretching and brisk walking.

My sister, Cameo, in fact, exercised right up until she delivered and when I visited her and the baby in the hospital, she looked healthier than 99 percent of the women on the streets. I was amazed at how energetic, rested, and fit she looked. It made me a lot less scared about having babies and losing my figure forever.

Experts agree that if you're already engaged in an exercise program, it's safe to continue with your doctor's approval. Pregnant women in high-risk categories may be advised to curb or modify their exercise programs.

Women who don't exercise at all during pregnancy naturally become progressively less fit as the months roll on. A marathon runner who quits exercise for nine months will have trouble running around the block after baby is born.

Most women in low-risk categories are encouraged to participate in aerobics, calisthenics, relaxation exercise, and Kegel exercises throughout their pregnancies.

Aerobic activities such as walking, jogging, cycling, and swimming actually aid pregnancy because they increase oxygen utilization for the mother and baby. Exercise also decreases the risk of hemorrhoids and fluid retention, and builds endurance and stamina so you won't tire as easily and will be able to withstand a lengthy labor.

In addition, it builds fat-burning muscle so you can eat a little more—all the pickles and (non-fat) ice cream you want!

Aerobic exercise also helps you sleep better, releases "happy hormones" (endorphins) that alleviate depression, helps relieve constipation, prevents varicose veins, increases muscle tone, and reduces backaches.

Light, rhythmic stretching exercises can improve muscle tone and posture and help prevent aches and pains that often accompany weight gain, while relaxation techniques—deep breathing, positive thinking, mental imagery—can ease anxiety that accompanies pregnancy. Kegel exercises—tensing and relaxing vaginal muscles, or what some women jokingly call the other pushups—can help tone and strengthen the vaginal and perineal area in preparation for delivery.

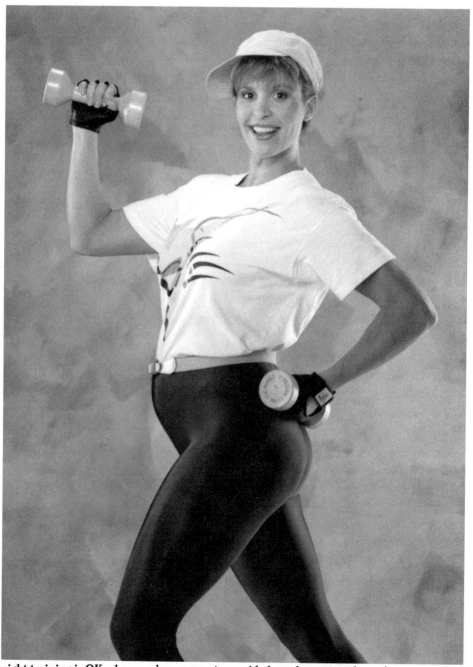

Even weight training is OK when you're pregnant, provided you have your doctor's permission and use very light weights.

SAFETY TIPS FOR MOTHERS-TO-BE

- Warm up first, start slow, finish as slowly as you started, and never overexert yourself.
- Drink lots of fluids and never work out on an empty stomach.
- Avoid exercise that causes your body to raise more than about 2 degrees Fahrenheit as it sends blood away from the uterus to the skin; stay out of hot tubs, saunas, and steam rooms for the same reason.
- Wear loose clothes that don't pinch or bind, and work out on indoor carpets.
- Stop exercising if you experience hip, back, pelvis, chest, or head pain, as well as cramps, stitches, dizziness, lightheadedness, or breathlessness.
- As for weight training, you can probably continue your program if it involves light weights, although your physician will undoubtedly discourage you from lifting anything very heavy.
- A few safe exercises for those in good shape include easy jogging up to 2 miles a day, cross-country skiing, cycling, aerobic classes, speedwalking, swimming in lukewarm water.
- Avoid running, horseback riding, scuba diving, sprinting, downhill skiing, outdoor cycling on slick pavement, and any contact sports.

THE DARK TRIAD; ANOREXIA, BULIMIA, AND EXERCISE ABUSE

Eating disorders—anorexia and bulimia—know no economic, social, or educational boundaries. One thing all sufferers share, however, is poor self-esteem. Eating disorders aren't about food as much as feelings, and food is the instrument of torture or deprivation.

Many women with eating disorders also abuse exercise to burn off every bite they eat. Exercise abuse is another disorder we'll discuss separately below.

Women typically develop these disorders in their teenage years, when the pressure to conform to societal standards of thinness peers out from every fashion magazine. If you ask me, these magazines should be burned as a health risk or be forced to carry a warning label: "Reading This Magazine Can Be Hazardous to Your Health."

Often left untreated, the disorder follows them into adulthood—often into menopause as well. They suffer silently and often alone, telling no one—not their families, friends, children, or lovers.

Meanwhile, the disorders play havoc with their physical and emotional health. Nutritional deficiencies resulting from near-starvation, can include hair loss, brittle bones, general fatigue, and a host of other health problems, while self-induced vomiting can lead to tooth loss and esophagus damage. Chronic yo-yo dieting drives a woman's metabolism to low levels and promotes even more starving, which in turn leads to more deficiencies. As you can see, it's a vicious circle and the emotional toil is equally great. While men are not off the hook, the vast majority of victims are women—in fact, the ratio is 9 to 1. (Surprised? Me neither!)

Ironically, most women who suffer eating disorders are overachievers—good little girls who from way back convinced themselves (usually with some help from parents or other family members) that no matter how hard they tried, they weren't smart or pretty enough. In the belief the only thing they can control is their bodies, they strive for perfection by starving, bingeing, or resorting to laxative abuse.

AS THIN AS A RAIL: ANOREXIA

Anorexia is defined by the American Psychiatric Association as an intense fear of becoming fat, which continues even as you lose weight. Many victims become completely emaciated. But when they look in the mirror, they still see a fat person looking back.

Victims typically lose about 15 percent of their normal weight and refuse to gain weight—sometimes even under medical supervision. They may hide food under their hospital beds, induce vomiting when the nurse leaves the room, or are found running stairs in the emergency stairwell to burn calories after they've removed their I.V.'s. Some signs of anorexia include intense fear of becoming fat, a distorted body image, hair loss, fine body hair that develops to keep the body warm, extreme sensitivity to heat and cold, playing with food at mealtime rather than eating it, a very low pulse rate, and an overly sensitive, nervous and anxious manner.

BINGE AND PURGE: BULIMIA

Bulimia, also called the binge-purge cycle and far more common than anorexia, is characterized by eating a large amount of food very quickly—high-fat foods such as ice cream, doughnuts, and cake are popular binge foods—then purging through self-induced vomiting, taking massive amounts of laxatives, or both. Victims typically become very depressed following a binge-purge cycle. Bulimia is so rampant on college campuses—as many as one in four women have suffered the disease at one time or another—that many universities have removed the doors from toilet stalls in womens' restrooms (good move!) to discourage secret purging.

Most bulimics are at normal weight or slightly above or below average, depending on where they are in their binge-purge cycle; rarely are they as stick-thin as anorexics. And while they may refuse to admit their problem, in their hearts they know they have one.

Telltale signs include frequent, secretive vomiting and subsequent loss of tooth enamel or teeth, frequent weight changes, puffy cheeks, dizziness and weakness, and secretive behavior around mealtime.

The good news is that women—including many famous women who seemed to have perfect lives—are coming out of the eating disorder closet in droves.

A great self-help guide for compulsive eaters is *Fat Is a Feminist Issue* by Susie Orbach, Berkley Books, New York, 1990.

NO MODEL ROLES HERE

By now the world is aware of Princess Diana's long-time battle with bulimia. Even if you rooted for Prince Charles when she left him, you have to credit Diana for her courage in speaking out about her disorder and for offering herself as a role model for other women.

Anyone who doubted the rumors concerning rampant eating disorders in the entertainment and modeling business became believers with the January 11, 1993, issue of *People Weekly* magazine. The cover portrayed three world-famous models with telling captions: Kim Alexis "starved herself for days," Carol Alt "fainted from hunger," and Beverly Johnson "binged and purged." All three said they learned the hard way that the only way to control their weight was by eating a healthful diet low in fat and high in carbohydrates combined with regular exercise. All three eat lots of pasta (carbs) and fresh vegetables, and go easy on the high-fat junk food.

OWN UP TO EATING DISORDERS

If you're bulimic, anorexic, or a binge-purger, or abuse laxatives, diuretics, or diet pills, the worst thing you can do is hide or try to deny your problem—the only person you're hurting is yourself.

Remember: these are diseases that primarily afflict perfectionists and overachievers—professional women with above-average intelligence and lofty goals comprise the majority of the ranks.

If you consider your recovery another goal—one which will ultimately let you lead a healthier and more productive life—it may help you finally admit your problem. Don't isolate yourself. There are a lot of women in your boat, and a lot of former sufferers anxious to help recover. For information about where to get help, contact these organizations:

ANRED (Anorexia Nervosa and Related Eating Disorders): Box 5102, Eugene, OR 97045; (503) 344-1144.

National Anorexic Aid Society: 5796 Karl Rd., Columbus, OH 43229; (614) 426-1133.

American Anorexia/Bulimia Association: 133 Cedar Lane, Teaneck, NJ 07666; (201) 836-1800.

A CRUCIAL PERIOD

Some women exercise so hard they stop having their periods, a condition called amenorrhea. Since regular menstruation requires a certain amount of calories, protein, and body fat their low body weights cannot sustain a period. Stress may also aggravate your normal cycle.

Amenorrhea is a warning sign that you are draining your body of energy; in fact, it is Mother Nature's way of preventing you from getting pregnant during a time when your body isn't up to the physical demands of it. Women who are very active in sports suffer a special type of amenorrhea called exercise-related amenorrhea or EAA.

According to studies by Barbara Drinkwater, Ph.D. at Pacific Medical Center at the University of California in San Francisco, this can lead to irreversible bone loss and the increased likelihood of developing osteoporosis in the long term, although symptoms may not appear until years later.

With lifestyle changes—reducing exercise by 10 percent and gaining at least four pounds—some women resumed menstruation without any other treatment and bone mass slowly increased. However, follow-up studies showed that their bone mass never returned to the levels of athletic women who menstruate regularly. The message? Never say diet—and don't overdo exercise. If you suffer from amenorrhea, seek medical care and be prepared to cut back on your workouts and gain two to ten pounds. If your period doesn't return in six to twelve months, you may be placed on hormone therapy.

EXERCISE ABUSE

If you feel compelled to exercise off every calorie you eat, or if your exercise program is crowding out everything else in your life—relationships, your job, free time—you should take a closer look.

While we'd be the first to applaud the merits of exercise, just like food, you can get too much of a good thing.

As with women who deprive themselves of food to seek perfection, exercise abusers overuse exercise to burn off every ounce before it becomes fat.

One of the first signs you're overdoing it is chronic fatigue (not to be confused with Chronic Fatigue Syndrome, a disease characterized by extreme tiredness and other symptoms), as well as insomnia, muscle soreness, frequent injuries, and a compulsion to exercise–rain or shine, in sickness or in health, or even if you're getting married in an hour.

Most abusers become isolated because their exercise programs require so many of their waking hours; often they become depressed and irritable and may suffer from amenorrhea.

Research shows too much exercise is harmful. If you suspect you're a victim of exercise abuse, nip it in the bud by taking these steps:

- Force yourself to take rest days and don't feel guilty about it. Too much training is counterproductive because it deprives your body of the rest time it needs to get stronger. Without rest, you put yourself at a higher risk of injuries and burnout.
- Alternate hard with easy workout days–one or two hard days with a moderate and easy day works well for many women.
- Don't equate your worth as a human being with how much you work out, how fast or well you perform, or what size clothing you wear.

If there's one thought we'd like to leave you with, it's that you're worth far more than the bathroom scale or the computer programs on your exercise machines could ever measure. Remember that the next time you're too tired to work out–take the day off! The track, treadmill, and dumbbells will still be there tomorrow. In the long run, you'll be better off physically for the break.

In addition, giving yourself a day off and the right to relax can be immensely empowering. Who knows? You may discover you're entitled to all sorts of things in life–not because you're perfect or trying to be, but just because you're you. Or as the ad puts it: "Why? Because I'm worth it!"

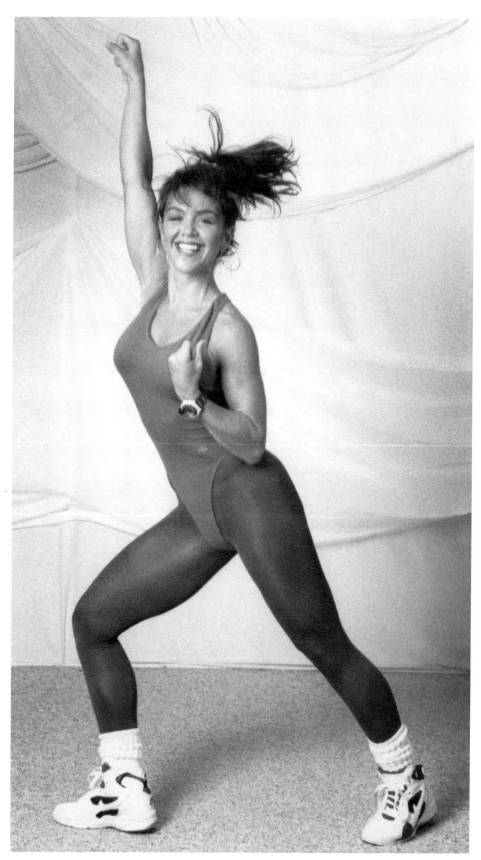

Michelle LeMay

Get fit with six-time Ms. Olympia
Cory Everson

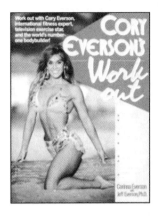 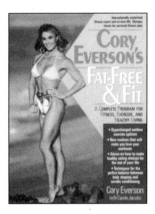

These books are available at your bookstore or wherever books are sold, or, for your convenience, we'll send them directly to you. Call 1-800-631-8571 (press 1 for inquiries and orders), or fill out coupon below and send it to:

The Berkley Publishing Group
390 Murray Hill Parkway, Department B
East Rutherford, NJ 07073

		U.S.	CANADA
____ Cory Everson's Workout	399-51684-0	$15.95	$20.95
____ Cory Everson's Fat-Free & Fit	399-51858-4	$15.00	$19.50

Subtotal $_____
Postage and handling* $_____
Sales tax (CA, NY, NJ, PA) $_____
Total amount due $_____

Payable in U.S. funds (no cash orders accepted). $15.00 minimum for credit card orders.

*Postage and handling: $2.50 for 1 book, $.75 each additional book up to a maximum of $6.25.

Enclosed is my   □ check   □ money order
Please charge my   □ Visa   □ MasterCard   □ American Express

Card #_____ Expiration date_____
Signature as on charge card_____
Name_____
Address_____
City_____ State_____ Zip_____
Please allow six weeks for delivery. Prices subject to change without notice.